C000162706

A Curious Herbal, Containing Five Hundred Cuts, of the Most Useful Plants, ... By Elizabeth Blackwell. To Which is Added a Short Description of ye Plants; ... of 2

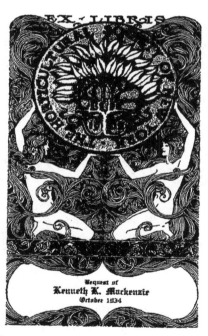

16

A CURIOUS HERBAL,

Containing

FIVE HUNDRED CUTS,

of the most useful Plants,

which are now used in the Practice of

PHYSICK.

Engraved on folio Copper Plates,
after Drawings, taken from

the LIFE.

By

Elizabeth Blackwell.

To which is added
a short Description of ẙ Plants,
and
their common Uses in PHYSICK.

Vol: I.

LONDON

Printed for JOHN NOURSE *at the Lamb without*
Temple Bar. MDCCXXXIX.

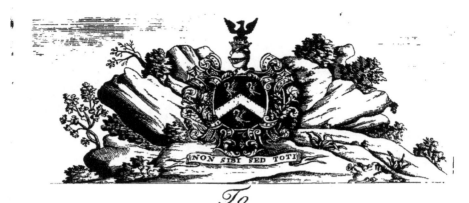

To

RICHARD MEAD M.D.

PHYSICIAN in Ordinary to his MAJESTY's and Fellow of the ROYAL COLLEGE of PHYSICIANS of London, and Fellow of the Royal Society. —

Sir

As the WORLD is indebted to the ENCOURAGERS of every Publick Good, if the following UNDERTAKING should prove such, it is but justice to declare who have been the chief PROMOTERS of it, and as you was the first who advis'd its PUBLICATION, and honour'd it with your NAME, give me Leave to tell the READERS how much they are in your Debt, for this WORK, and to acknowledge the Honour of your FRIENDSHIP.

I am

Chelsea ye 14th of July 1737

Sir with great Respect your most obliged humble Servant
Elizabeth Blackwell

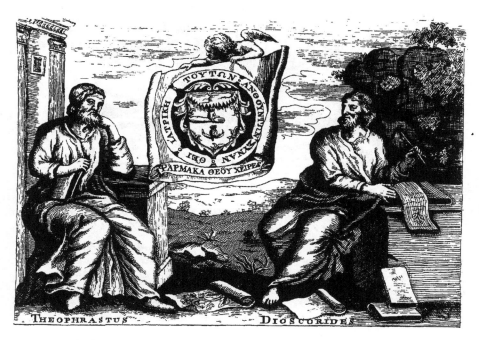

THEOPHRASTUS   DIOSCORIDES

Dat Comitiis Censoriis ex Ædibus Collegii nostri Die primo Julii 1737

Imagines hasce Plantarum Officinalium per Dominam ELISABETHAM BLACKWELL *delineatas, æri incisas & depictas, iis qui Medicinæ Operam dant, perutiles fore judicamus* ——

THOMAS PELLET, *Præs*

HENRICUS PLUMPTRE,
RICHARDUS TYSON, } *Censores*
PEIRCIUS DOD,
GULIELMUS WASEY,

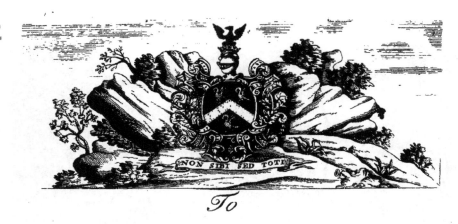

NON SIBI SED TOTI

To

This UNDERTAKING *was honoured with the following Publick*
RECOMMENDATION *by the Underwritten Gentlemen*

London October 1 1735

*We whose Names are underwritten, having seen a considerable Number
of the* DRAWINGS *from which the* PLATES *are to be Engraved,
and likewise some of the* COLOUR'D PLANTS, *think it a
Justice done the* PUBLICK *to declare our Satisfaction with them,
and our good Opinion of the Capacity of the Undertaker.*

R MEAD, MD	IA DOUGLAS, M.D.	IOSEPH MILLER
G.L TEISSIER, MD	IAMES SHERARD, MD	ISAAC RAND
ALEX.ᴿ STUART, MD.	W CHESELDEN.	ROB. NICHOLLS

Les PERSONNES *soussignées ont bien voulu faire à l'*AUTEUR
de cet OUVRAGE *l'honneur de lui donner leur*APPROBATION
de la maniere Suivante

Londres ce 1 Octobre, 1735

Nous soussignés, ayant vû un assés grand nombre des DESSIENS
sur lesquels on doit graver les PLANCHES, *de même que
quelques unes des* PLANTES ENLUMINÉES, *avons trouvé le
tout si bien* EXECUTÉ *que nous avons conçu une* IDÉE *avant-
ageuse de la Capacité de l'Auteur; & nous avons tout lieu de croire
que le* PUBLIC *recevra cet Ouvrage favorablement*

R MEAD, MD	IA DOUGLAS MD	IOSEPH MILLER
G.L TEISSIER, MD.	IAMES SHERARD, MD	ISAAC RAND
ALEXᴿ STUART, MD	W CHESELDEN	ROB NICHOLLS

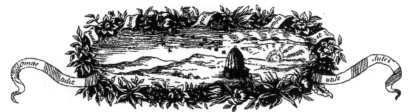

INTRODUCTION,

The Undertaker, being desirous to make this Work more useful to such as are not furnished with other Herbals, is resolved (for their Sake) to give a short Description of each Plant, the Place of Growth, and Time of Flowring with its common uses in Physick, chiefly extracted from Mr Joseph Miller's Botanicum Officinale with his Consent; and the ordinary Names of the Plant in different Languages

---

Plate 1 Dandelion, or Piss-a-bed. Dens Leonis.

1 The Leaves of this Plant lie on ÿ Ground, the Pedikels or Pipes on which the Flowers grow are about six or eight Inches high, and the Flowers yellow. The Root grows about a Finger thick, and eight Inches long, full of a white bitter Milk.
2 It grows almost every where in Fallow Ground, & flowers most Months in the Year.
3 The Root & Leaves are used, as cooling, aperative, provoking Urine, & strengthening ÿ Stomach and are much eat as a Sallad in the Spring
4 Greek, Αφακα. Latin, Dens Leonis, Taraxacum. Spanish, Diente de Leon Italian, Dente di cane and Piscia al letto French, Dens de Lyon, or Pisse en lict German, Pfaffenblatt & Bunnichstopff Dutch, Papercruyt

---

Plate 2 Red, Wild, or Corn Poppy. Papaver rubrum

1 This Plant grows to be 2 Foot high, the Leaves are a Willow-green, & the Flowers Scarlet
2 It grows in most Corn-fields, and flowers in Iune and Iuly
3 The Flowers of this Poppy are cooling, incline to sleep, & much used in inflamatory Fevers. Officinal Preparations from it are, ÿ simple Water, ÿ Syrup, ÿ Conserve of ÿ Flowers & ÿ Tincture
4 Greek, Μηκων εριας Latin, Papaver, rubrum, erraticum, rhoeas Spanish, Amapolas or Papoulla Italian, Papavero salvaticho French, Pavot sauvage, or confanons German, Clapper Rosen, or Corn Rosen Dutch, Rooden huel

---

Plate 3 Mullein or Hig-Taper Verbascum or Tapsus barbatus

1 It grows to be six Foot high, the Leaves are a light Willow-green, & the Flowers a pale Yellow
2 They grow in Highways and Commons, and flower in Iuly
3 The Leaves are used for Coughs, Pains in ÿ Breast and Collic-Pains, & outwardly in Fomentations, and are thought a specific against the Piles Dioscorides recommends a Decoction of the Root is good for the Tooth ach
4 Greek, Φλομος Latin, Verbascum or Tapsus barbatus Spanish, Gordolobo or Verbasco Italian, Tasso barbasso French, Bouillon German, Beyß Bullcraut Dutch, Wolle kruyt

---

Plate 4 Garden Cucumber. Cucumis sativus

1 This Plant trails on ÿ Ground, the Leaves are a Yellow green, & the Flowers a pale Yellow
2 It is raised from ÿ Seed yearly, & flowers, & bears Fruit for several Months in the Summer
3 The Seed is used for the Stone, Strangury, heat of Urine, burning Fevers and Plurisies Dioscorides says, the Fruit chears decayed Spirits, and recommends the Leaves boiled with Wine, and mixed with Honey as a Cure for the Bite of a Dog
4 Greek, Σικυς ημερος Latin, Cucumis sativus, vulgaris Spanish, Cogombro Italian, Cocomero French, Cocombre German, Cucumera Dutch, Concomeren

No 1.

Plate 1

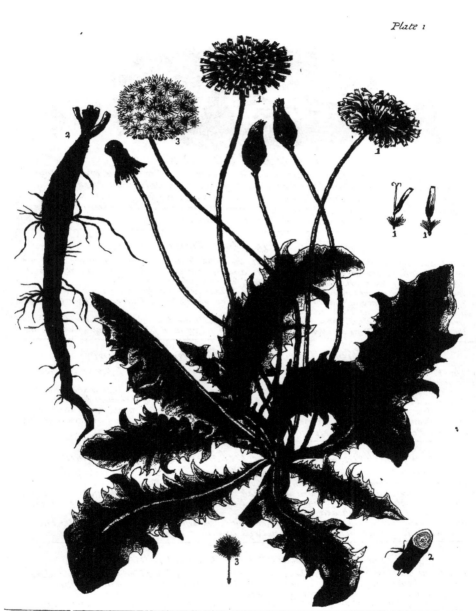

Dandelion

Eliz. Blackwell delin sculp et Pinx

{1 Flower}
{2 Root}
{3 Seed}

Dens Leonis
Taraxacum

Plate 2

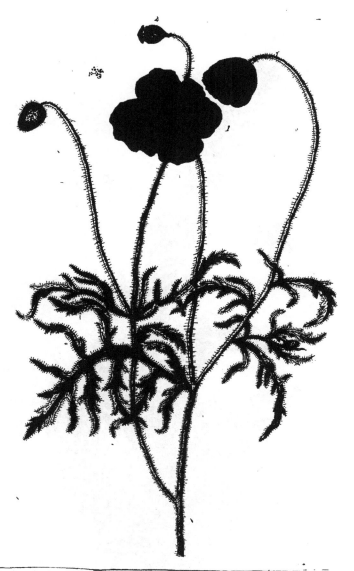

Red Poppy

Eliz Blackwell delin sculp et Pinx

1 Flower
2 Fruit
3 Seed

Papaver

rubrum
erraticum
rhœa

Plate 3

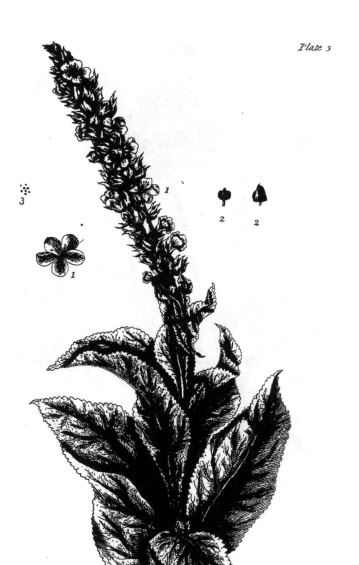

1

1

2   2

3

Mullein

Hog Taper

Eliz Blackwell delin sculp et Pinx

{1 Flower

{2 Fruit

{3 Seed

Verbascum

Tapsus barbatus

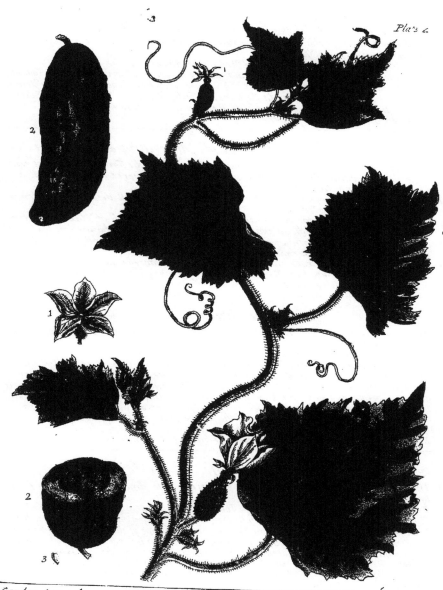

Pla'z 6.

Garden Cucumber

Eliz. Blackwell delin. Sculp. et Pinx.

1 Flower
2 Fruit
3 Seed

Cucumis Sativus

Plate 5 Shepherd's Purse. Bursa Pastoris.

1 The lower Leaves lie flat upon the Ground, the Stalk grows about a Foot high, and the Flowers are White

2 It grows among Rubbish Banks and Walls, and flowers all the Summer

3 This Plant is esteemed cooling, restringent, incrassating, & good in all sorts of Fluxes & spitting of Blood, bleeding at y Nose, the too great Flux of y Catamenia, violent Floodings, & bloody Urine.

4 Greek. Latin, Bursa Pastoris, or Thlaspi fatuum Italian, Bursa Pastoris French Bourse a Pasteur, or Bourse de Berger German, Sectelcraut, Secfel, or Zeschellcraut Dutch, Borse kens cruyt

---

Plate 6 Wild Tansie, or Silver-weed. Argentina or Potentilla

1 This Plant creeps upon the Ground, emitting Fibers from the Joints, by which it roots in the Earth and spreads, the Leaves are a light green covered as it were with a silver Down, and the Flowers a yellow

2 It grows in most barren Ground where Water has stood all the Winter & flowers commonly in May or Iune

3 The Leaves are restringent and vulnerary, good to stop all kinds of Fluxes & preter-natural Evacuations, to dissolve coagulated Blood, to help those who are bruised by Falls, outwardly it is used as a Cosmetic to take off Freckles, Sun-burn and Morphew and is good in restringent gargarisms

4 Greek. Latin, Argentina, Potentilla Tanacetum agreste Italian Potentilla French L'Argentine sauvage, or Tanesie sauvage German, Genserich, Grensich, or Gensing Dutch, Silvercruyt

---

Plate 7 Rue Ruta.

1 The Leaves are a Willow-green, and the Flowers yellow, the Stalks grow about two Foot high

2 It is planted in Gardens, and flowers in Iune and Iuly

3 The Leaves and Seed are used being esteem'd alexipharmic, good against all infectious and pestilential Diseases, and all kind of Fevers, it eases Disorders of the Head, Nerves, Womb convulsion and Histeric Fits, the Collick, Weakness of the Stomach and Bowels. it repells Poison, and cures the Bite of venemous Creatures and mad Dogs It is an Ingredient in the Aqua Brion comp and the Aqua Theriacalis The officinal Prepara tions are the simple Water, Conserve of the Leaves, and an Oil by Decoction

4 Greek, Πηγανον Latin, Ruta & Ruta hortensis major Spanish, Aruda Italian, Ruta French, Rut German, Rauten or Beincraut Dutch, Ruyte

---

Plate 8 Wild Rose or Briar Rose Rosa Canina

1 The Leaves are a darker green than the Garden-rose, and the Flowers are some times white, but oftener a pale Red

2 It grows in Hedges, & flowers in Iune & Iuly The Hips are fit to gather the latter End of September On the Stalks of this Bush y Bedeguar grows which is a reddish green spongy hairy Excrescence, made by small Ichneumon Flies See Ray's Catalogue of the Plants about Cambridge, p 140

3 The Flowers of this Rose are thought more restringent than y Garden Some look upon them as a specific for y Excess of y Catamenia The Pulp of y Hips strengthens y Stomach cools the Heat of Fevers is pectoral good for Coughs spitting of Blood & y Sturry The Seed is good against y Stone and Gravel The Bedeguar is said to have the same Virtues The officinal Preparation is the Conserva Cynosbati

4 Greek, Κυνοσβατος, βοδον αγριον οι Κυνόρροδον, Latin Rosa Canina or Rosa Sylvestris French, Le Rosier or l'Eglantier sauvage german Bilderosen or Hetrosen Dutch Eglantier

Plate 5

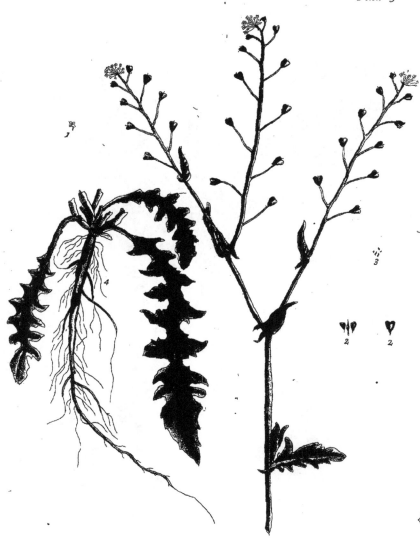

Shepherds Purse

Eliz Blackwell delin sculp et Pinx

1 Flower
2 Fruit
3 Seed
4 Root

Bursa Pastoris

Plate 6

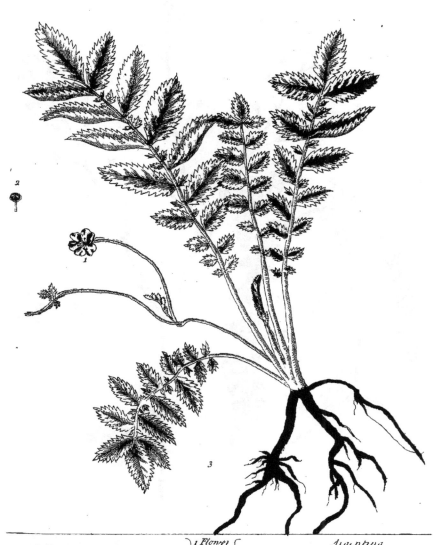

Wild Tanſie

Eliz. Blackwell delin. sculp. et Pinx

1 Flower
2 Fruit
3 Root

Argentina
Potentilla

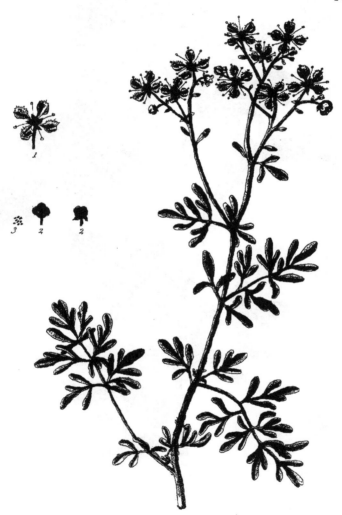

Plate 7

Rue

Rue

1 Flower
2 Fruit
3 Seed

Plate 8

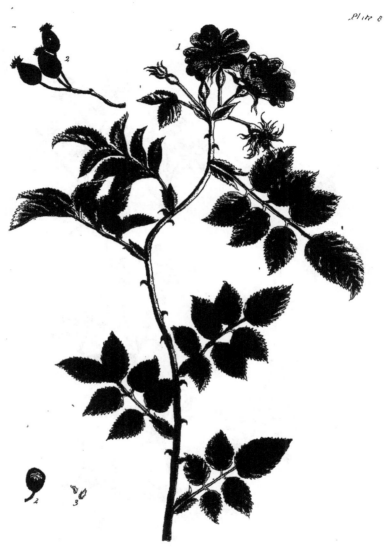

Wild Rose

Eliz Blackwell delin sculp et Pinx

1 Flower
2 Fruit
3 Seed

Rosa

Plate 9 Wood Sage. Salvia agrestis or Scorodonia

1 This Plant grows to be two Foot high, its Leaves are greener and broader than the Garden Sage, the Flowers are yellow, with purple Stamina
2 It grows in Hedges and bushy Places, and flowers in July and August
3 It is esteemed good for the Gout, Rheumatism, Scurvy & Dropsy, provoking Urine & the Menses, it is an excellent vulnerary Plant, preventing Mortifications & Gangreens.
4 Greek Σκόρδιον Latin, Scordium, Salvia agrestis, Scorodonia Spanish, Scordio Italian, Scordio French, Chamaraz German, Bafferbatenig, or Knoblochfcraut.

Plate 10 Sage Salvia.

1 It is planted in Gardens, the Leaves are sometimes a hoary Green, & sometimes a reddish Purple, the Flowers are a bluish Purple, and grows about 18 Inches high
2 It grows best in dry sharp Ground, and flowers in May and Iune.
3 The Leaves and Flowers are used, as good for all Diseases of the Head and Nerves, they are also diuretic, and good for Obstructions of Urine, and much used in all Sorts of Fevers, in Tea or Poffet Drink
4 Greek, Ἐλελιοφακ⊚ Latin, Salvia, and Salvia hortensis major. Spanish, Salvia and Salva Italian, Salvia. French, Saulges German, Salben Dutch.

Plate 11 White Lilly. Lilium album

1 The Lilly grows about four Foot high, the Flowers are white, with yellow Apices in the middle
2 It is planted in Gardens, and flowers in Iune and Iuly
3 The Flowers and Roots are used chiefly in external Applications, they are softning and anodine, good to diffolve and ripen hard Tumours and Swellings, and to break Impofthumations Matthiolus recommends the Oil, made of the Flowers, as good for all Pains of ye Joints & contracted Nerves The officinal Preparation is ye Oleum Liliorum
4 Greek, Κείνον, λέιειον Latin, Lilium album, and Lilium album flore erecto Spanish, Azucena, and Lirio blanco Italian Giglio branco French, Lis German, Zilgen and Gilgen Dutch. Lelie.

Plate 12 Stinging Nettle Urtica.

1 This Nettle grows to be two Foot high, the Leaves are of a lighter Green than the Roman Nettle the Flowers are a dull Yellow
2 The Nettle grows every where in too great Plenty, and flowers for several Months in the Summer
3 The Roots, Leaves and Seed are used as cooling and restringent, the Juice is thought good for all kinds of inward Bleedings Haemorrhagies and Fluxes A Tent dipt in it stops the Bleeding of the Nose or Wounds The Root is esteemed diuretic, and a Specific for the Iaundice The Seed is recommended for Coughs shortnefs of Breath, and Obstructions of the Lungs
4 Greek, Ἀκαλύφη or Ἀκαλήφη Latin, Urtica urens and urens maxima Spanish Ortiga Italian, Ortica French, Ortie German Bellschoder Romisch Teffel Dutch.

No 3

Plate 9

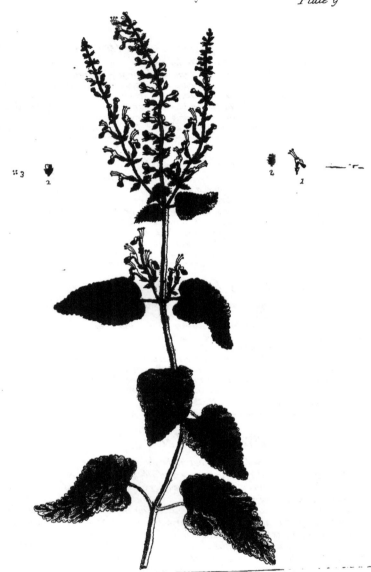

Wood Sage

1 Flower
2 Fruit
3 Seed

Scorodonia

Salvia silvestris

Blacknell delin. sculp et Pinx

Plate 10

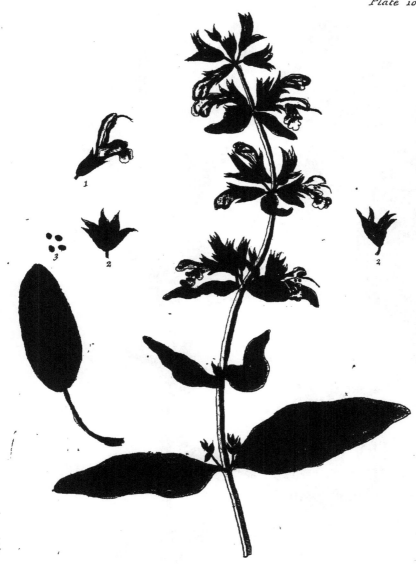

Sage   1 *Flower*   *Salvia*
Eliz. Blackwell delin sculp et Pinx   2 *Fruit*
3 *Seed*

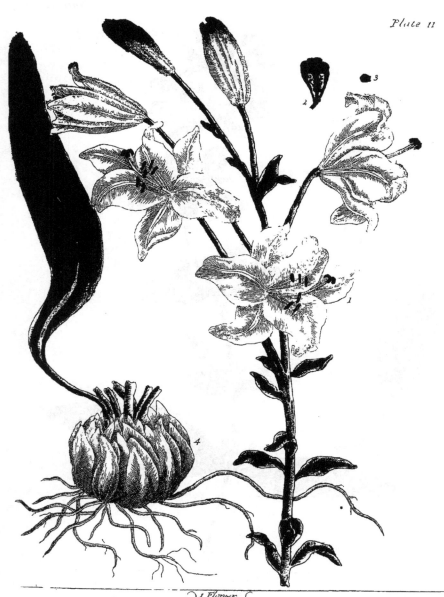

Plate 11

White Lilly   1 Flower   Lilium album
: Black W Li... ulp et Pi...   2 Fruit
                               3 Seed
                               4 Root

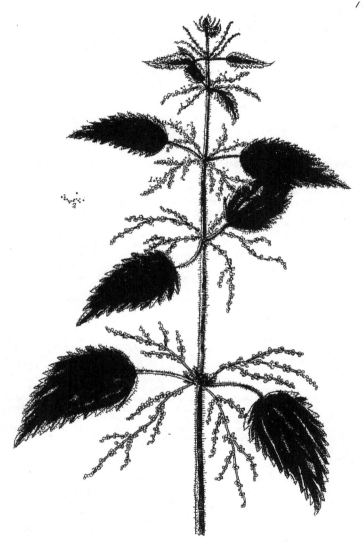

Stinging Nettle

Blackwell delin: sculp: et Pinx:

{ 1 Flower
{ 2 Seed

Urtica

Plate 13 Jasmine, or Jessamine. *Jasminum or Jasminum album*

1. This Shrub shoots forth long slender green Twigs, which would lie on y.º Ground if they were not supported; the Flowers of the common Jasmine are white
2. It is planted with us in Gardens, and flowers for several Months in the Summer
3. The Flowers are the only Part used Schroder commends them as good to warm & relax the Womb, to heal any Schirrhi therein, and to facilitate the Birth, and also for a Cough and Difficulty of breathing The Oil made by Infusion of the Flowers is used in Perfumes Matthiolus thinks that the Ointment made of Jasmine by the Ancients was not that Jasmine which we have now
4. Greek, Latin, Jasminum or Jasminum album or Gelsiminum Italian, Gelsimino French, Jasmin German, Beielreben. Dutch

Plate 14 Narrow-leaved Plantain, or Ribwort. *Plantago angustifolia, or Quinquenervia*

1. It grows to eight or nine Inches high, the Leaves have five Nerves which run quite thro' them from the Root, the Flowers are of a light Umber colour with white Apices
2. It grows in Fields and Meadows, and flowers mostly in May and Iune, altho' you may find some of it in Flower most Months of the Summer.
3. It is cold dry and binding, good in all kind of Fluxes and Haemorrhages as spitting or vomiting of Blood, bleeding at the Nose, the Excess of the Catamenia or Lochia It stops ye involuntary making of Urine, eases its Heat & Sharpness, & the Gonorrhea, & stops the bleeding of Wounds The officinal Preparation is, the simple distilled Water
4. Greek, Ἀρνόγλωσον μακρὸν or πλατάνελζο Latin, Plantago angustifolia & Quinquenerva Italian, Piantagine longa or Lanciola French, Plantain German, Spigiger Wegrich. Dutch,

Plate 15 St John's Wort *Hypericum.*

1. This Plant grows to be two Foot high, the Leaves when held up against the Light appear full of small Holes, the Flowers are a bright Yellow, with a great Number of Apices & Stamina, which being bruised between ye Fingers emit a bloody Iuice
2. It grows in Hedges and among Bushes, and flowers in Iune and Iuly
3. St John's Wort is accounted aperative, detersive, diuretic, alexipharmic, good in tertian and quartan Agues, destroys Worms, and is an excellent vulnerary Plant A Tincture of ye Flowers in Spirit of Wine is commended against Melancholy & Madness Outwardly it is of great Service in Bruises, Contusions & Wounds, especially in die nervous Pai ts The officinal Preparations are, the simple and compound Oil
4. Greek, Ύπερικον Latin, Hypericum or Hypericum vulgare Spanish, Corajoncillo Italian, Hyperico and Perforata, or Herba di S Giovanni French. Millepetius or Trucheran. German, Sanct Iohannicraut Dutch

Plate 16 Fox-Glove *Digitalis.*

1. It grows to be three Foot high, the Leaves have a little Down upon them y Flowers are red, spotted with white, and grow all on one side of the Stalks
2. Fox-Glove grows in Hedges and Lanes, and flowers in Iune and Iuly
3. This Plant is but rarely used inwardly, being a strong Emetic working with Violence upwards and downwards de Parkinson extolls a Decoction of it in Ale, with Polipody Roots, as an approved Medicine for ye Falling Sickness The late Doctor Hulse commends ye Ointment made of the Flowers and May Butter, for scrophulous Ulcers, which run much diet ing them with the Ointment and purging two or three Times a Week with proper Pu ge The officinal Preparation is the Unguentum digitalis
4. Greek, Latin, Digitalis, or Digitalis purpurea Spanish, Italian French la Digitale German, Dutch,

Plate 11

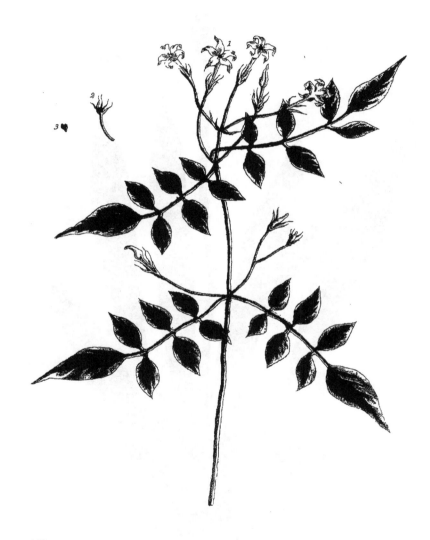

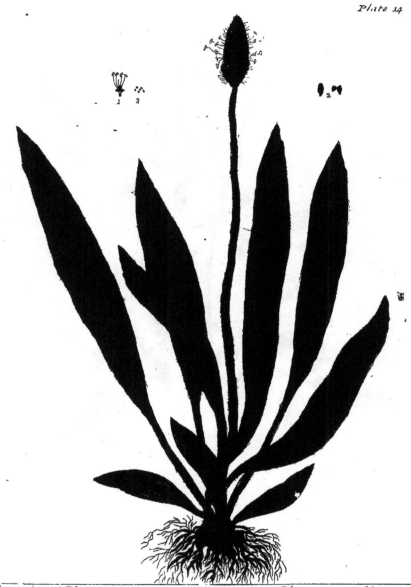

Plate 14

Narrow leaved Plantain   1. Flower   Plantago angustifolia
    Ribn ort   2. Fruit   Quinquenervia
Eliz Blackwelldelin sculp et Pinx   3. Seed

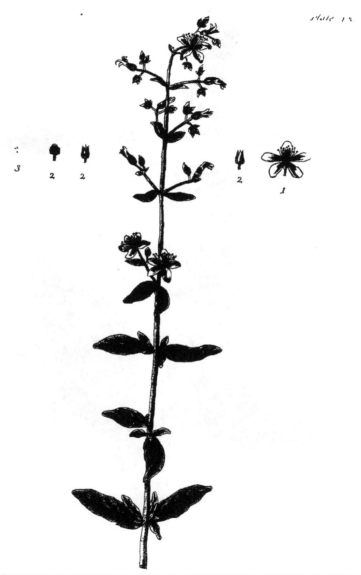

Plate 15

3 2 2 2 1

St John Wort

Das Blaknei   { 1 Flower
                       2 Fruit
                       3 Seed   Hypericum

Plate 11

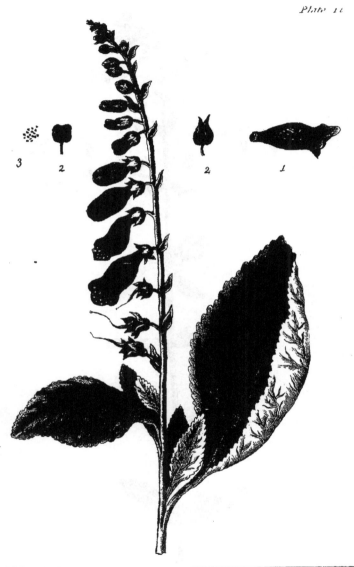

3   2   2   1

Fox glove   1 flower   Digitalis
4 = Blackwell delin sculp et Pinx   2 fruit
                              3 seed

Plate 17 Wormwood. Abfinthium vulgare.

1 It grows to be three Foot high, the Stalks are hoary full of a white Pith, y Leaves are a Willow-green above, & a light hoary underneath, the Flowers are yellow
2 It grows in Lanes and waste Places, and flowers in July and August
3 The Leaves & Tops are used, they purge Melancholy Humours, provoke Urine, restore an Appetite that is lost by Drinking They are good against the Diforders of y Stomach, vomiting & Surfeits, they strengthen the Viscera, kill Worms, & are of service in Dropfies, Jaundice, tertian & quartan Agues In all y above cafes it is infused in Water, Ale or Wine. A Cataplafm of the green Leaves beat up with Hog's Lard was commended to M.r Ray by D.r Hulse as a good external Remedy against y swelling of the Tonfils & Quinzy See Rays Cat Plantarum Officinal Preparations are, a simple Water; a greater and a lesser compound Water, a simple and a compound Surup; an Oil by infufion, and decoction, and Oil by Dyftillation, an Extract; a fixt Salt.
4 Greek, Aψίνθιον. Latin, Abfinthium vulgare or Ponticum Spanish, Affentos or Alofna. Italian, Affenzo or Affenta. French, Aluyné or Abfince German, Wermut. Dutch, Alfem.

Plate 18 Yarrow or Milfoil Millefolium.

1 The Stalks grow about eighteen Inches high, and are fomewhat hairy, the Flowers are white, and grow on the Tops of the Branches in flat Umbels
2 It grows in most Fields, and flowers in June and July
3 The Leaves are efteemed cooling, drying, binding, serviceable in all kinds of Haemorrhages, as fpitting or vomiting Blood, bleeding at the Nofe, Dyfentery the two great Flux of the Menfes, violent flooding, cooling and tempering its immoderate Sharpnefs, it is good in a Gonorrhea, Strangury, Heat of Urine, when applied outwardly it is of Service against Ruptures & ftaunches y bleeding of Frefh Wounds
4 Greek, Στρατιωτης χιλιοφολλ☉ μεγας Latin, Millefolium terreftre vulgare, or vulgare Flore albo Spanish, Millhogas yerva Italian, Millefoglio French, Millefueille German, Garben Dutch, Duyfruid-blad.

Plate 19. The Garden Bean Faba major, or major hortenfis.

1 The Garden Bean grows to be three or four Foot high, the Leaves are a pale Green, and the Flowers white, with two black Spots in them
2 It is fown in Gardens, and flowers in May, and the Beans are ripe in June or July
3 The Water diftilled from y Flowers is used by many as a Cofmetic, & that from the Pods is accounted good for y Wind & Gripes in Children. Diofcorides fays, y Meal made into a Cataplafm removes y Swellings in Women's Breafts which are occafioned by the Milk, he alfo recommends it mixt with Rofes, Time, & y white of an Egg, as good for purging all watery Rheums from y Eyes, & mixed with Wine as good for y Web & bloodfhot of the Eyes The Meal given inwardly is efteemed good for a bloody flux The officinal Preparations are, the Aqua Florum et Siliquarum Fabarum.
Greek, Κυαμ☉ Latin, Faba major, or Faba major hortenfis Spanish, Havas Italian, Fava. French, Fave German, Bonen Dutch, Roomfe, or Bocre-Boonen

Plate 20 Meadow Trefoil or Clover Grafs Trifolium vulgare.

The Leaves are a pale Green, and the Flowers purple fpotted with white, the Stalks grow to be eighteen Inches high
It grows in moft Fields and Meadows, and flowers in May or June
The Leaves & Flowers are used as drying, binding, good for all kind of Fluxes y Strangury & heat of Urine, made into a Cataplafm with Hog's Lard they are reckoned good for Tumours & Inflammations Matthiolus fays a Decoction of y Whole Plant in Flower, ftops y Whites in Women
Greek, Τρίφυλλον Latin, Trifolium vulgare Spanish, Italian, Trifoglio French, Troisfueille German, Biefenclee Dutch, roode Klaaveren
No 5

Plate 17

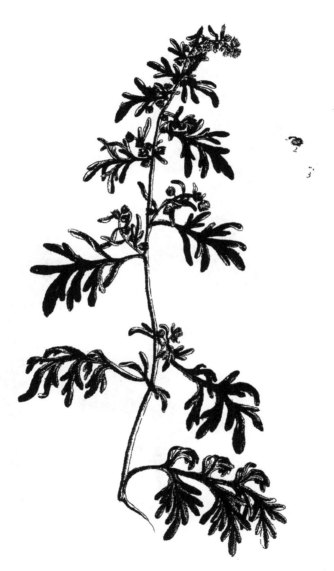

2

3

Wormwood

Eliz Blackwell del sculp

{ 2 Fruit
{ 3 Seed }

Absinthium

Plate 18

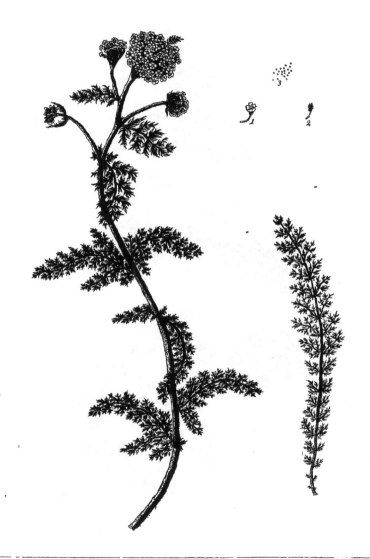

Yarrow

1 *Flower*
2 *Fruit*
3 *Seed*

Millefolium

Plate 19

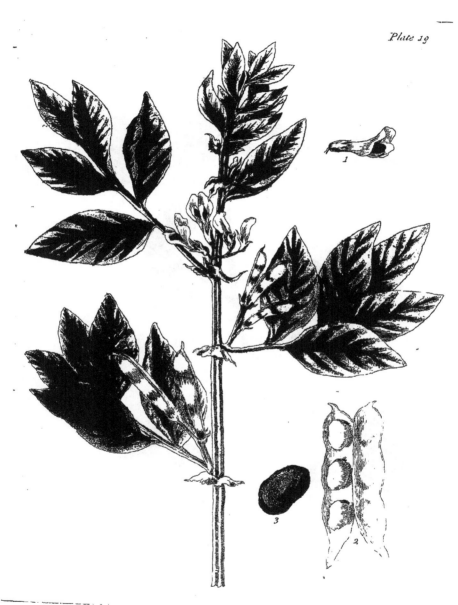

The Bean
bI z Blackwell dihn sulp et Pin

1 Flower
2 Fruit
3 Seed

Iala

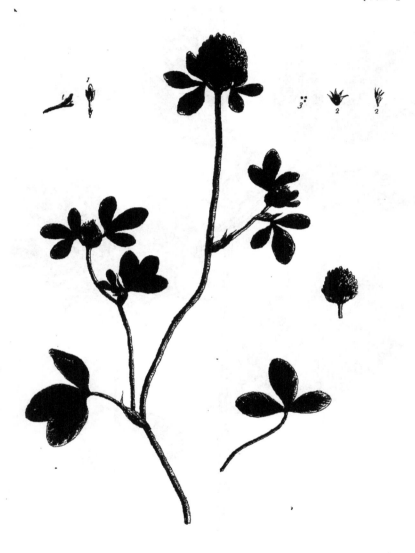

Plate 2

Purple Trefoil
Clover Grass
az Blackwell delin sculp et Pinx.

} 1 Flower {
} 2 Fruit {
} 3 Seed {

Trifolium vulgare

Plate 21 ## Agrimony Agrimonia

1 This is the Eupatorium of Dioscorides, Galen, & the ancient Greeks, it grows about two Foot high, having several ringed hairy Leaves of a pale green Colour, and yellow Flowers
2 It grows in Hedges, and the Borders of Fields, and flowers in June and July
3 Agrimony is esteemed cleansing and purifying for the Blood, strengthning ye Liver, and good in all Diseases arising from the Weakness thereof, as the Dropsy, Jaundice &c Matthiolus recommends it with white Wine as an excellent Cure for the Strangury and bloody Water Riverius extols ye Powder of ye dried Leaves for the Incontinence of Urine It is likewise a vulnerary Plant, & put in Wound-Drinks, & outwardly used in Baths & Fomentations
4 Greek, Ευπατοριον. Latin, Agrimonia. or Eupatorium Græcorum Spanish, Agramonia Italian. Agrimonia French, Agremoine German Aderineng Dutch, Agremonie

Plate 22. Common Mallow Malva vulgaris

1 Mallows grow to be three Foot high, the Stalks are somewhat hairy, & the Leaves are a yellowish Green, ye Flowers are a bright reddish Purple strip'd with a deep Purple
2 It grows commonly by Way-sides, and flowers for most Months in the Summer.
3 This is one of the five emollient Herbs, being Loosening, cooling & Molifying A Decoction of the Leaves, sweetned with Syrup of Violets, & drank now and then to the Quantity of a Quarter of a Pint, keeps the Body soluble assuages choleric Humours, allays the heat & sharpness of Urine, eases the Stone & Gravel, and provokes Urine A Cataplasm made of the Leaves, eases the smart of the Place that is stung by Bees or Wasps. Where Marsh Mallows are not to be had this may supply the Place
4 Greek, Μαλαχη Latin, Malva & Malva vulgaris, or agrestis Spanish, Malvas Italian, Malba, or Malva French, Malve German, Pappel Dutch, Kaassecruud

Plate 23 Garden Cress Nasturtium Hortense

1 It grows to be eighteen Inches high, the Leaves are a bright Green, & the Flowers white
2 It is sown in Gardens yearly, and flowers most Months in the Summer
3 The Leaves are much used as a Sallad, their warmth being good to help the coldness of others mixed with them They are esteemed good for the Scurvy, Dropsy, Palsy and Lethargy A Cataplasm of the Leaves with Hogs Lard cures scald Heads the Seed helps the Scurvy and Dropsy, and swelling of the Spleen, and opens Obstructions in the Female sex, and prevents the falling off of the Hair
: Greek, Καρδαμον Latin, Nasturtium Spanish, Nasturtio, and Malpica Italian Nasturtio and Agretto French, Cresson de Jardins, and Nasitort German, Garten cress Dutch, Thuyn-Kersse

Plate 24 Self-Heal. Prunella or Brunella

This Plant grows to be a Foot high, the Leaves are of dark Green and the Flowers Purple
It grows in Meadows and pasture Grounds, flowering all the latter Months of the Summer
It is used for all Inflammations and Ulcers in the Tongue, Jaws and Throat either the Juice or a strong Decoction, as also for inward Bleedings & making of Bloody Water.
Greek, Ευπατοριον Latin Prunella or Prunella vulgaris Spanish Agramonia Italian, Consolida minore. French, Agremoine German, Brunellen & Adermenie Dutch Brunelle

Plate 21

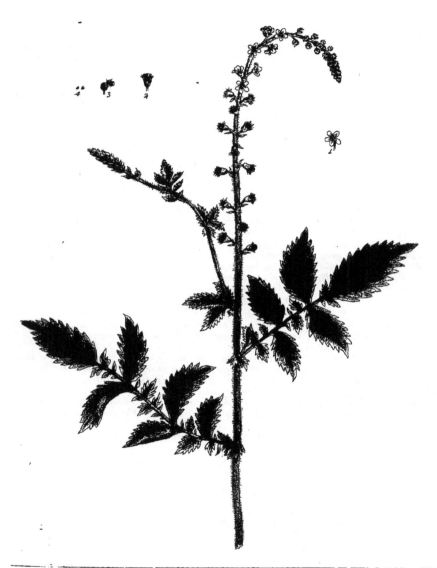

Agrimony

Blackwell delin. sculp et Pinx

{ 1 Flower
{ 2 Fruit
{ 3 Fruit cut
{ 4 Seed

Agrimonia
Eupatorium graveum

Plate 22

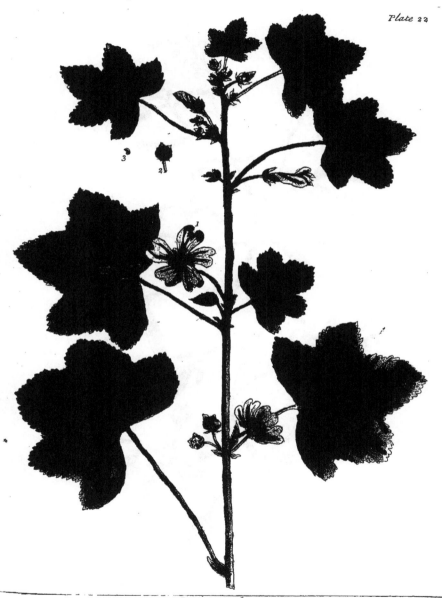

Mallow

Eliz.Blackwell delin sculp et Pinx

1 *Flower*
2 *Fruit*
3 *Seed*

Malva

Plate 40

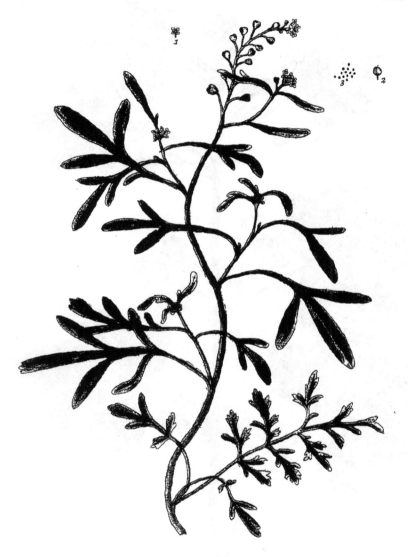

Crefs
Garden Crefs
Eliz Blackwell delin sculp et Pinx

} 1 Flower {
} 2 Fruit {
} 3 Seed {

Nasturtium
Nasturtium hortense

Plate 7

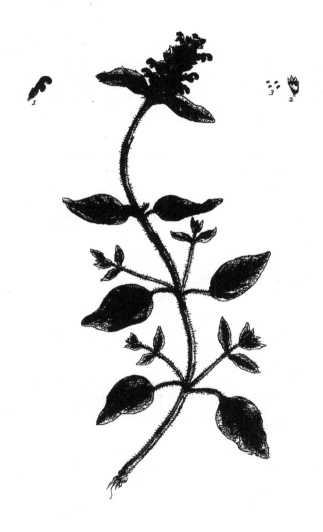

Self Heal

Eliz Blackwell delin sculp et Pinx

1 Flower
2 Cup
3 Seed

Prunella
Brunella

Plate 25 *Wood-Bind or Honey-Suckle Caprifolium or Periclemenum*

1 This Shrub grows to the thickness of eight or ten Inches in circumference, shooting out long slender Stalks, which twist about every thing they meet with, the Leaves are a bluish green, and the Flowers a pale red which are succeeded by Berries of a deeper Red

2 It grows in most Hedges, and flowers the greatest part of the Summer

3 The Leaves are sometimes put into Gargarisms for sore Throats Some commend a Decoction of them for a Cough and the Ptysick, and to open Obstructions of y Liver & Spleen The Oil, made by infusion of y Flowers, is accounted healing & warming, good for the Cramp & Convulsions of y Nerves Matthiolus recommends the Leaves & their Juice as good in the Ointments that are used for Wounds in the Head, and Ulcers in the Legs

4 Greek, Περικλύμενον Latin, Caprifolium, & Periclemenum Spanish Madreselva Italian, Vincibosco French, Vincitosse German, Bergslatt Dutch, Geytenblad & Mammetges-kruyd

---

Plate 26 *Lark's-Spur. Delphinium, or Consolida regalis*

1 It grows to be a Yard high, the Leaves are a dark green, and the Flowers commonly a fine blue, but sometimes a Purple

2 It is sown every Year in Gardens, and flowers most part of the Summer

3 This is esteemed a vulnerary Plant, of a healing Nature Matthiolus says it cures the Rheums and Inflammations of the Eyes, mixed with Honey & drank with sweet Wine it removes the sharpness of Urine It likewise closes up fresh Wounds, and heals Ulcers

4 Greek, Δελφίνιον Latin, Delphinium or Consolida regalis Spanish. Italian, Consolida reale French Pie d'Allouette German Rittersporea Dutch Ridderspoin

---

Plate 27 *Balm Melissa*

1 This Plant grows to be three Foot high, the Stalks are square the Leaves a light yellow green, and the Flowers white

2 It grows only in Gardens here and flowers in July and August

3 The whole Herb is used, and esteemed cordial, cephalic, good for Disorders of the Head and Nerves, chears the Heart, cures its Palpitation, prevents Fainting, Melancholy, Hypochondriac and Hysteric Disorders, resists Putrefaction, and is of great service in malignant and contagious Distempers, outwardly applied it helps the stinging of Bees and Wasps The officinal Preparation is, the Simple Water

4 Greek, Μελισσόφυλλον Latin, Melissa or Melissophyllum Spanish Torongil or Herva cidrein Italian, Melissa French, Melisse & Poncirade German, Melissen Mutterkraut Dutch confilie de greyn

---

Plate 28 *Hedge Mustard Erysimum*

1 It grows to be two Foot high, the Leaves are a yellow green, & y Flowers a pale Yellow

2 Hedge-Mustard grows commonly by Way-sides, and on Banks, and flowers most part of the Summer

3 This Plant is hot dry, opens & attenuates, by its warming Quality, it dissolves thick and slimy Humours in y Lungs, helps a Cough and shortness of Breath It is much recommended against an habitual Hoarseness, to recover y Voice Riverius praises a Decoction of it in Wine, as a good remedy for y Colic The officinal Preparation is, the Syrupus de Erysimo

4 Greek, Ἐρύσιμον Latin Erysimum Spanish, Rinchaon French Velar or Tortelle Italian Erisimo or Irion. German, Hederich & Wilder Stuff Dutch, Steen-Raket

No 7

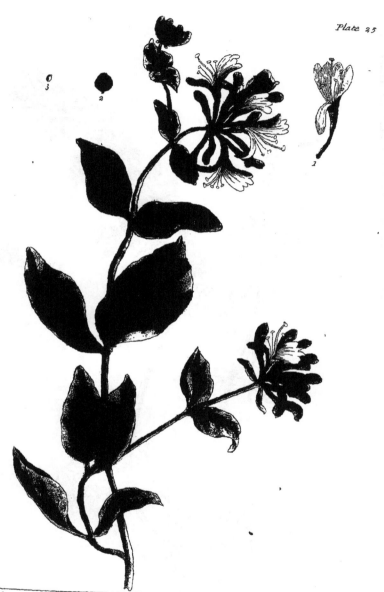

Plate 25

Honey Suckle
Wood Bind

E. Blackwell delin: sculp et Pinx

{ 1 Flower
2 Fruit
3 Seed }

Periclymenum
caprifolium utriusq.

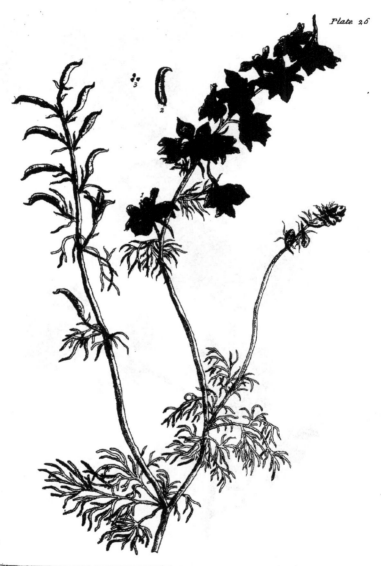

Plate 26

Lark Spur

Eliz Blackwell delin sculp et Pinx

1 Flower
2 Fruit
3 Seed

Consolida regalis
Delphinium

Plate 2

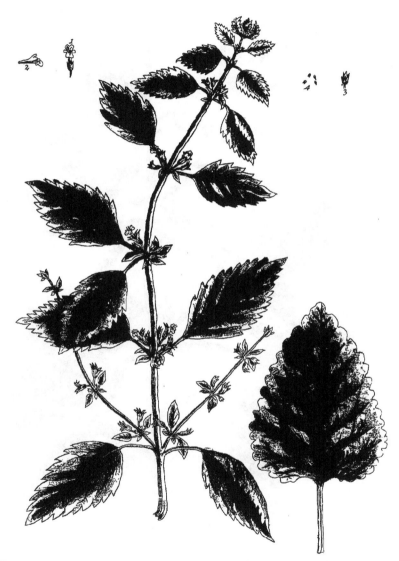

Balm

Eliz Blackwell delin sculp et Pinx

{ 1 Flower with its Cup
{ 2 Flower Separate
{ 3 Cup
{ 4 Seed

Melissophyllum

Plate 28

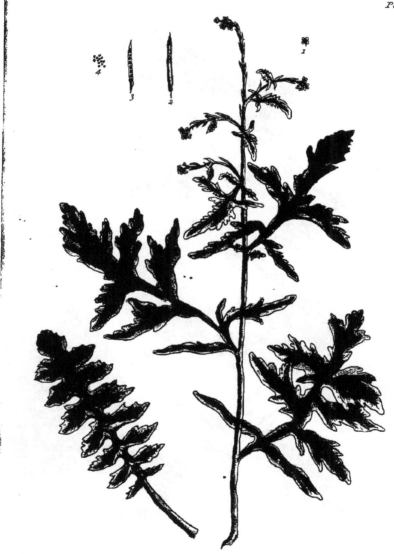

Hedge Mustard

Eliz Blackwell delin sculp et Pinx

1 Flower
2 Pod
3 Middle Membrane
4 Seed

Erysimum

Plate 29 *White Mustard. Sinapi album.*

1 The Stalks grow to be two Foot high, and are hairy, the Leaves are a light Green, and the Flowers a bright yellow

2 It grows wild in dry Banks, and the Edges of Fields, and flowers in Iuly

3 The Seed provokes an Appetite, strengthens the Stomach and helps Digestion Dioscorides recommends the Iuice mixed with Water and Honey as good to gargle the Throat with, and help Women who are troubled with the Mother; a Cataplasm of Figs and the Iuice is good for the Lethargy, by laying it on the Head, shaved, till the place grows red, & the same Cataplasm laid on ye Hip eases the Sciatica. The Seed he recommends as good in Plaisters to soften ye Scabs of the Head

4 Greek, Σίνπωι έτερον. Latin, Sinapi album or alterum Spanish, Mostaxa blanco Italian, Senape or Senauro salvatico French, Seneve blanc. German, Gelder Senff Dutch, Wit Mostard-Zaat

---

Plate 30. *Sow Thistle. Sonchus asper.*

1 It grows about two Foot high, the Leaves are a bright Green, and the Flowers a pale yellow

2 This Sow-Thistle grows commonly on Banks, and flowers in May and Iune

3 The Leaves are of the same Nature with those of the Dandelyon, being aperative and diuretic, and good for the Gravel and stoppage of Urine Matthiolus says the Roots and Leaves when young are much used in Italy in Sallads, & recommends the Milk of the Stalk in Wine as good for an Asthma, & the distempers of the Ear, when boiled with Oil Galen recommends ye Leaves to be chewd for an offensive Breath

4 Greek, Σόγχος, Σόγχος Latin, Sonchus asper Spanish, Serraya or Serralha Italian, Soncho, Cicerbita French, Latteron German, Bilder Hasentol or Gausdistel Dutch, Gonse-distel

---

Plate 31 *Crow-foot Ranunculus pratensis repens*

1 This Plant grows to be a Foot high, the Stalks and Leaves are somewhat hairy, the Flowers are a shining bright Yellow

2 It grows in most Fields, and flowers in May

3 Crow foot is caustic and may be used to draw Blisters, where Cantharides cannot be had, but they must not ly on too long, for fear of ulcerating the Part The Bavarians extol the distilled Water from the Leaves of the bulbous sort, or the Leaves infused in Brandy, as an excellent Remedy against the Plague

4 Greek, Βαρράχιον & σελινοράγριον Πλατυφυλλος Latin, Ranunculus pratensis Spanish Yerva belida Italian, Ranoncolo or Pie Corbini French, Grenoillette or Bassinet German, Hanen Fuss Dutch, S. Anthonis Raapje

---

Plate 32 *Water-Mint Mentha aquatica or Sisymbrium*

1 It grows to be 8 Inches high ye Stalks are hairy, & ye Flowers a red Purple and ye Leaves a reddish Green

2 It grows in Ditches and Watery-places, and flowers in Iune and Iuly

3 This Mint is rather hotter than ye Garden Mint being carminative expelling Wind out of the Stomach & helping ye Collic, it opens Obstructions of ye Womb and procures the Catimenia The Iuice dropd into the Ears is good to ease their Pain & help Deafness Dioscorides recommends the Leaves boiled in Water as good to stop a Red humor or Tumor

4 Greek Σισούμβριον Latin Mentha aquatica or Sisymbrium Spanish Berva . . . Italian, Sisimbrio French, German, Dutch Bosch water Munt

No 8

Plate 29

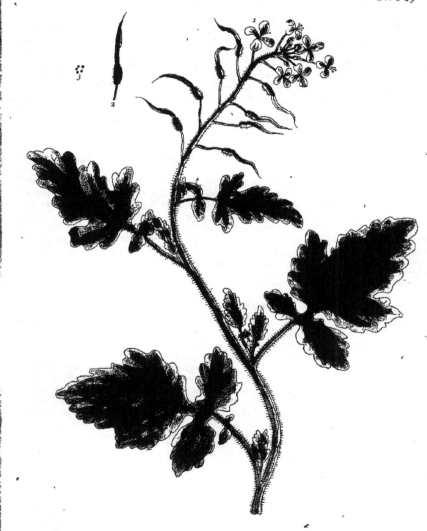

White Mustard

Eliz Blackwell delin sculp et Pinx

1 Flower
2 Fruit
3 Seed

Sinapa album

Plate 30

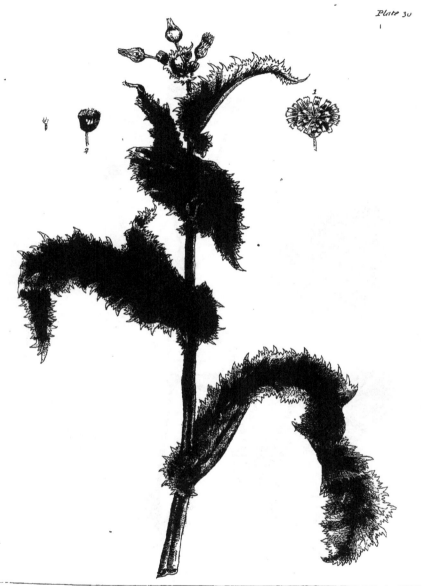

Prickly Son Thiſtle

Eliz Blackwell delin sculp et Pinx

1 *Flower*

2 *Cup*

Sonchus asper

Plate 31

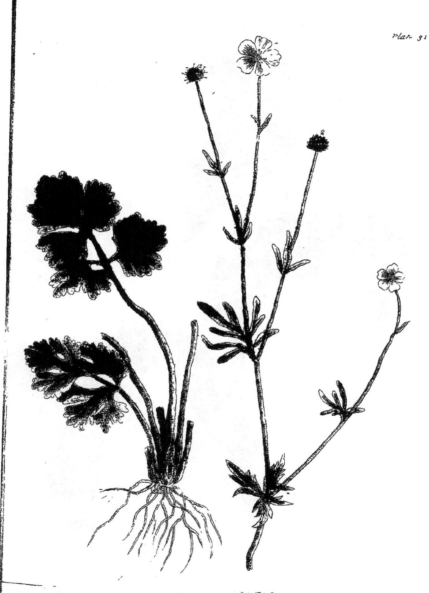

Crow foot

Eliz Blackwell delin sculp et Pin

1 Flower
2 Fruit

Ranunculus

Plate 32

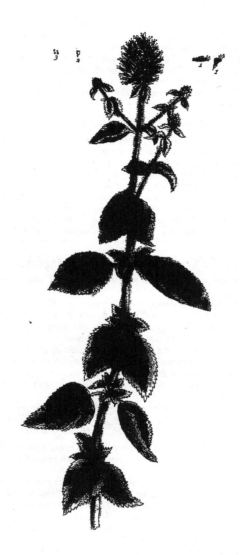

Water Mint

Eliz Blackwell delin sculp et Pinx

{ 1 Flower
2 Cup
3 Seed }

Mentha aquatica
Sisymbrium

Plate 33 *White-Archangel or Dead-Nettle Lamium album or Urtica mortua.*

1 The Stalks grow to be a Foot high, the Leaves are a dark Green and the Flowers White

2 It grows by Hedges, and flowers in April and May

3 The Flowers are accounted a Specific against the Fluor albus, and are frequently made use of in a Conserve or Decoction for that purpose, which is to be continued for some time Some recommend this Plant as of great use against the King's-Evil, and all scrophulous Swellings The officinal Preparation is, the Conserve of the Flowers

4 Greek, Ταλιοψις Latin, Lamium album, or Urtica mortua Spanish, Ortica muerta Italian, Ortica fetida, or Ortica morta French, Ortie. German. Daubneffel. Dutch Dood Netelen

---

Plate 34 *Woody Night-Shade, or Bitter=Sweet. Solanum lignosum, or Dulca mara*

1 This Species of Night-Shade has many long ash-coloured Branches, that climb up upon any thing it grows near to, the Leaves are a deep Green, and the Flowers Purple.

2 It grows in most Hedges & watery Places, and flowers in May and Iune.

3 The Leaves and Twigs are used, and are commended by some against the Dropsy, Iaundice, and King's-Evil. Parkinson says it purges violently enough Prevotius in his Medicina Pauperum, commends it as a kindly Evacuator of Bile. Dioscorides commends the Berries as good to take Spots out of the Skin.

4 Greek, Άμπελος άγρία Latin, Solanum lignosum & Dulca mara Spanish, Italian, Vite salvatica French, Morele German. Ielengerje heber Dutch. Groote winde.

Plate 35 *Broad-leaved Plantain. Plantago latifolia, or Septinervia.*

1 The Stalks of this Plantain grow to be eight Inches high, the Flowers are a whitish Colour.

2 It grows by Way-sides and Meadows, and flowers in May

3 Plantain is cold, dry, and binding, usefull in all kinds of Fluxes and Haemorrhages, as spiting & vomiting of Blood, bleeding at the Nose, the Excess of the Catamenia or Lochia. It is likewise esteemed good for the involuntary making of Urine, its Heat and Sharpness, & the Gonorrhea, it helps to stop ý bleeding of Wounds & consolidate their Lips. The officinal Preparation is the Simple distilled Water

4 Greek, Άρνόγλωσσον Latin, Plantago latifolia, or Septinervia. Spanish, Lhantem or Tamehagem Italian, Piantagine or Centinervia French, Plantain German. Megrich. Dutch, Weeg bree.

Plate 36. *Borrage. Borrago, or Buglossum*

1 It grows to be 18 Inches high, the Leaves are a grass Green, and the Flowers Purple

2 It grows frequently as a Weed in Gardens, and is often found wild near Houses and upon Walls, and flowers in Iune.

3 The Leaves are esteemed cordial comforting the Heart, preventing Faintness & Melancholy. The Tops are much used in Wine & Cool-Tankards They are accounted Alexipharmic, and good in malignant Fevers The Flowers are one of the four cordial Flowers. The officinal Preparation is the Conserve of the Flowers. Matthiolus recommends the whole Plant distilled, as good for ý Inflammations of the Eyes, whether inwardly or outwardly applied

4 Greek, Βούγλοσσον Latin, Borrago or Buglossum Spanish, Borraja, Borrazenes, Borrajes Italian, Borragine French, Borrache German. Burretsch Dutch, Bernaasje

Plate 33

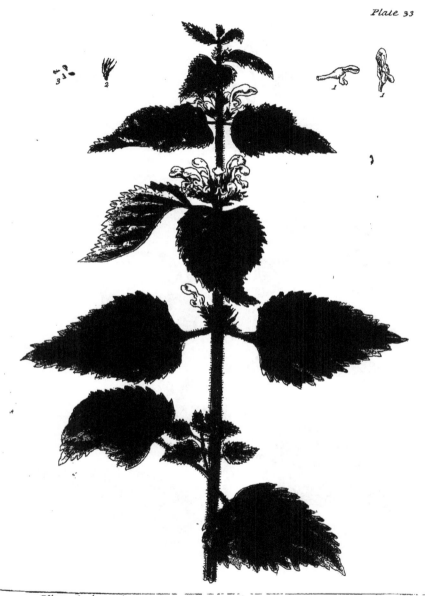

White Archangel
Dead Nettle

Eliz Blackwell delin sculp et Pinx

1 Flower
2 Cup
3 Seed

Lamium album
Urtica mortua

Plate 34

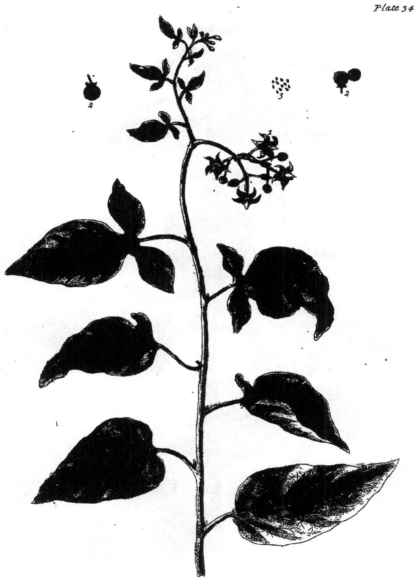

Woody Night-shade
Biter-sweet
Eliz Blackwell delin sculp et Pinx

} 1 Flower {
} 2 Fruit {
} 3 Seed {

Solanum lignosum
Dulca mara

Plate 35

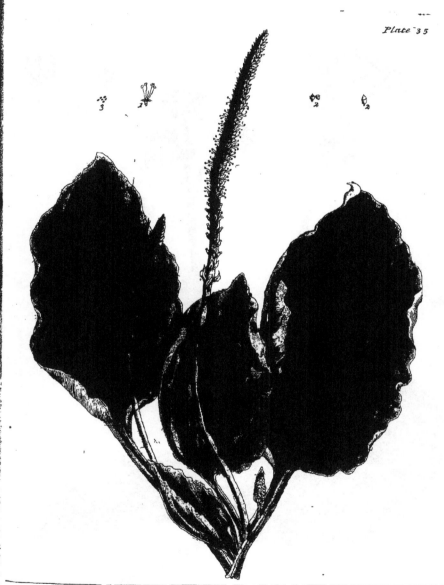

Plantain

Eliz Blackwell delin. culp et Pinx

1 Flower
2 Seed Vesell
3 Seed

Plantago
Septinervia.

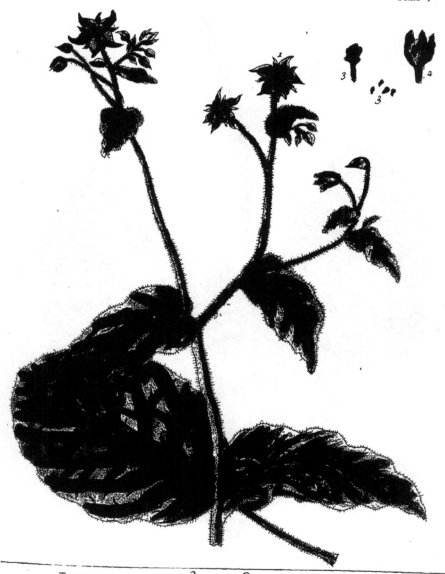

Plate 1

Borrage

Eliz Blackwell delin sculp et Pinx

{ 1 Flower
2 Calex
3 Seed }

Borago

Plate 37 **White Briony. Bryonia alba or Vitis alba.**

1 The Stalks of this Briony climb up to a great Height in the Hedges, the Leaves much resemble those of a Vine, the Flowers are a whitish green Colour

2 It grows in Lanes and Hedges, and flowers in May and Iune

3 The Root is a strong Purger of serous watery Humours, which it does both upwards and downwards, & is esteemed good for ÿ Dropsy. Gout. Epilepsy, Palsy & hysteric Disorders Doctor Sydenham commends it very much in cases of Madness The Faecula is much of the same Nature, but something Weaker The officinal Preparations are the Aqua Brioniae comp or the Hysteric Water, and the Faecula Brioniae.

4. Greek, Ἄμπελος λευκή Latin, Bryonia alba, or Vitis alba. Spanish, Neuza, or Anorca. Italian, Brionia, or Zucca salvatica French, Colubrine or Couluree german, Stictvurk or Zeufelsturbss. Dutch, Wilde Wyngaarde

Plate 38 **Great White Bindweed. Convolvulus major albus, or Smilax laevis.**

1 It runs up to a great height when it has any thing to twist about, the Leaves are a willow Green, and the Flowers white.

2 This Plant grows in most Hedges, and flowers all the latter end of the Summer

3 The Root of the Great White Bindweed is somewhat cathartic Prevotius in his Medicina Pauperum reckons it a gentle Evacuator of the Bile Camerarius doubts whether this be the Smilax laevis of the Antients

4 Greek, Σμίλαξ λεια Latin, Convolvulus major albus, or Smilax laevis Spanish, Correquela major Italian, Vilucchio maggiore French, Liset or Campanetre. German, Binden Dutch, Groote Winde

Plate 39 **Clivers or Goose Grass. Aparine.**

1 This is a creeping Plant that grows annually from the Seed, the Stalks, Leaves and Seed are rough, and the Flowers are white

2 It grows in most Hedges, and flowers for several Months in the Summer

3 The whole Plant is used, & is esteemed moderately cooling & drying. good to sweeten ÿ Blood, It is also accounted vulnerary, & of Service in ÿ Kings-Evil, for which some give the Iuice as a great Secret It is likewise diuretic, and helps the Stone and Gravel This is one of those Herbs which are commonly put into Spring Porridge as good for the Scurvy

4 Greek, Ἀπαρίνη. Latin, Aparine Spanish, Italian, Aparine, or Speronella French, German, Klebcraut. Dutch, Kleef-kruyd

Plate 40 **Wheat, & Bearded Wheat. Triticum, & Triticum aristatum**

1 The Wheat without Awns or Beards is that which grows most common in England, some call the Bearded Wheat Dugdale Wheat

2 It is sown commonly in Autumn and reaped the Iuly or August following

3 This Grain is reckon'd more nourishing than any other Grain for Bread A Poultice made of it boiled in Milk eases Pains, and ripens Tumours & Imposthumations A piece of Bread, toasted and dip'd in Wine, is good to stop Vomiting, by applying it to the Stomach. The Bran is used in Cataplasms, and applied hot in Bags for Pains in the Sides. There was formerly kept in the Shops an Emplastrum de Crusta Panis

4 Greek, Πυρός. Latin, Triticum or Triticum aristatum Spanish, Trigo Italian. Grano or Tormento French, Fourment German, Beissen Dutch, Tarraw.

No 10.

Plate 37

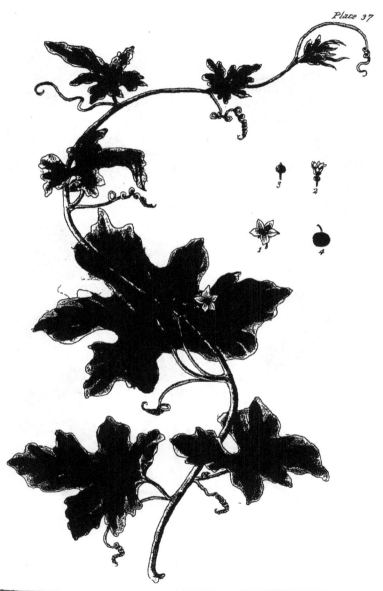

Bryony

Eliz Blackwell delin sculp et Pinx

1 Flower
2 Fruit & Flower
3 Fruit Green
4 Fruit Ripe

Bryonia alba
Vitis alba

Plate 38

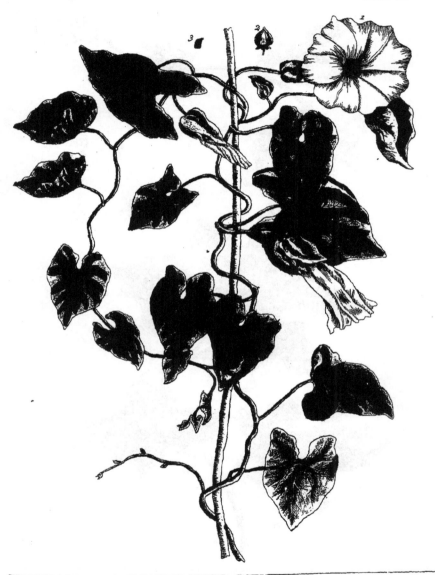

Great Bindweed
Eliz Blackwell delin sculp et Pinx

1 Flower
2 Fruit
3 Seed

Convolvulus major albus
Smilax Levis

Plate 39

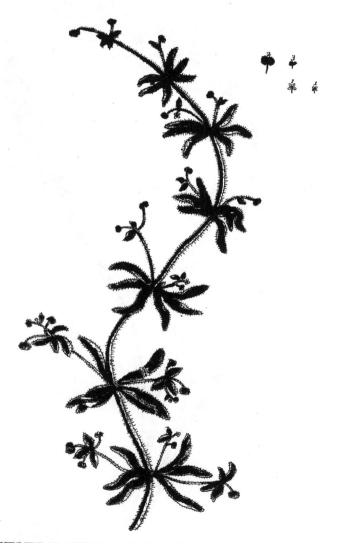

Clivers
Goose Grafs
Eliz Blackwell delin sculp et Pinx

{ 1 Flower
{ 2 Fruit
{ 3 Seed.

Aparine

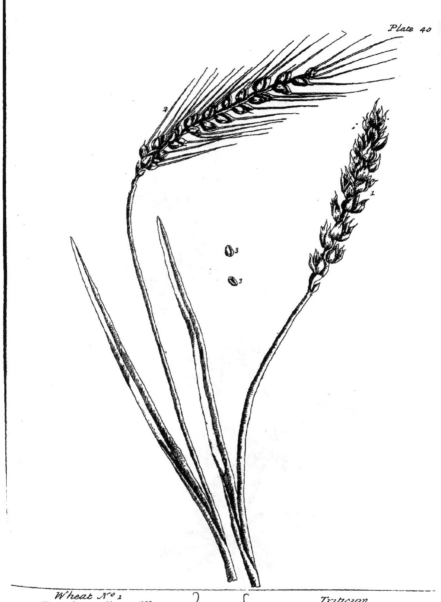

Plate 40

Wheat N.º 1
Bearded Wheat N.º 2
Elizz Blackwell delin sculp et Pinx

} 3 Seed {

Triticum
Triticum aristatum

Plate 37 White Briony Bryonia alba or Vitis alba

1 The Stalks of this Briony climb up to a great Height in the Hedges, the Leaves much resemble those of a Vine the Flowers are a whitish green Colour
2 It grows in Lanes and Hedges and flowers in May and Iune
3 The Root is a strong Purger of serous watery Humours, which it does both upwards and downwards, & is esteemed good for ÿ Dropsy Gout Epilepsy, Palsy & hysteric Disorders Doctor Sydenham commends it very much in cases of Madness The Faecula is much of the same Nature, but something Weaker The officinal Preparations are the Aqua Bryoniae comp or the Hysteric Water, and the Faecula Bryoniae
4 Greek, Ἄμπελος λευκή Latin, Bryonia alba, or Vitis alba Spanish, Neura or Anorca Italian Bryonia, or Zucca salvatica French, Colubrine or Couluree German, Stictwurk or Zeufellturlss Dutch, Wilde Wyngaarde

---

Plate 38 Great White Bindweed Convolvulus major albus, or Smilax laevis

1 It runs up to a great height when it has any thing to twist about, the Leaves are a willow Green, and the Flowers white
2 This Plant grows in most Hedges, and flowers all the latter end of the Summer
3 The Root of the Great White Bindweed is somewhat cathartic Prevotius in his Medicina Pauperum reckons it a gentle Evacuator of the Bile Camerarius doubts whether this be the Smilax laevis of the Antients
4 Greek, Σμίλαξ λεῖα Latin, Convolvulus major albus, or Smilax laevis Spanish, Correguela major Italian, Vilucchio maggiore French Liset or Campanetre German, Binden Dutch, Groote Winde

---

Plate 39 Clivers or Goose Grass Aparine

1 This is a creeping Plant that grows annually from the Seed, the Stalks Leaves and Seed are rough, and the Flowers are white
2 It grows in most Hedges, and flowers for several Months in the Summer
3 The whole Plant is used & is esteemed moderately cooling & drying, good to sweeten ÿ Blood. It is also accounted vulnerary, & of Service in ÿ Kings Evil, for which some give the Iuice as a great Secret It is likewise diuretic, and helps the Stone and Gravel This is one of those Herbs which are commonly put into Spring Porridge as good for the Scurvy
4 Greek, Ἀπαρίνη Latin Aparine Spanish Italian Aparine or Speronella French, German, Klebcraut Dutch Kleef-kruyd

---

Plate 40 Wheat, & Bearded Wheat Triticum, & Triticum aristatum

1 The Wheat without Awns or Beards is that which grows most common in England, some call the Bearded Wheat Dugdale Wheat
2 It is sown commonly in Autumn and reaped the Iuly or August following
3 This Grain is reckon'd more nourishing than any other Grain for Bread A Poultice made of it boiled in Milk eases Pains, and ripens Tumours & Imposthumations A piece of Bread toasted and dipd in Wine is good to stop Vomiting by applying it to the Stomach The Bran is used in Cataplasms, and applied hot in Bags for Pains in the Sides There was formerly kept in the Shops an Emplastrum de Crusta Panis
4 Greek, Πυρός Latin Triticum or Triticum aristatum Spanish, Trigo Italian Grano or Formento French Fourment German, Beissen Dutch Tarraw

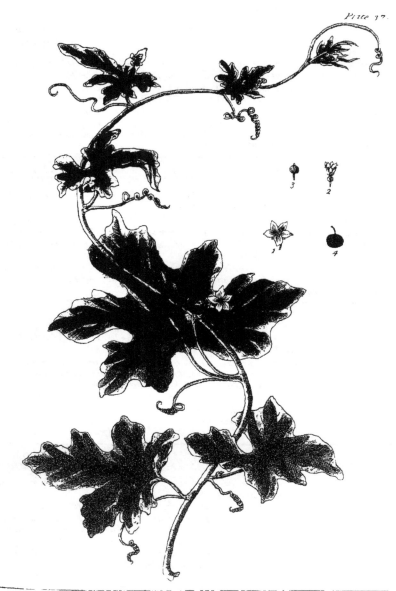

Plate 37.

Bryony

by Bl. knell delin sculp et Pinx

1 Flower
2 Fruit & Flower
3 Fruit green
4 Inch to

Bryonia alba
Vitis alba

Plate 38

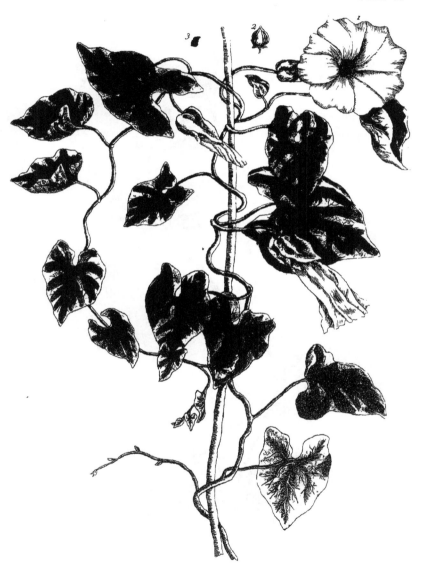

Great Bindweed

1 Flower
2 Fruit
3 Seed

Convolvulus major albus
    Inatis Lorii

Plate 30

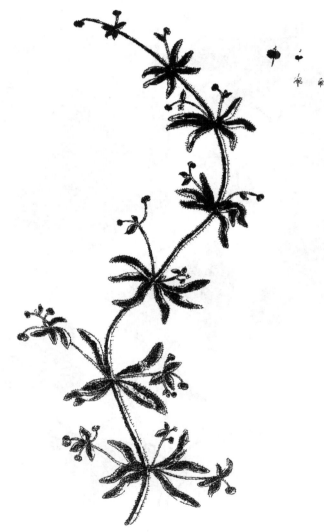

The Bleriot ... Flower 2 Fruit 3 Seed

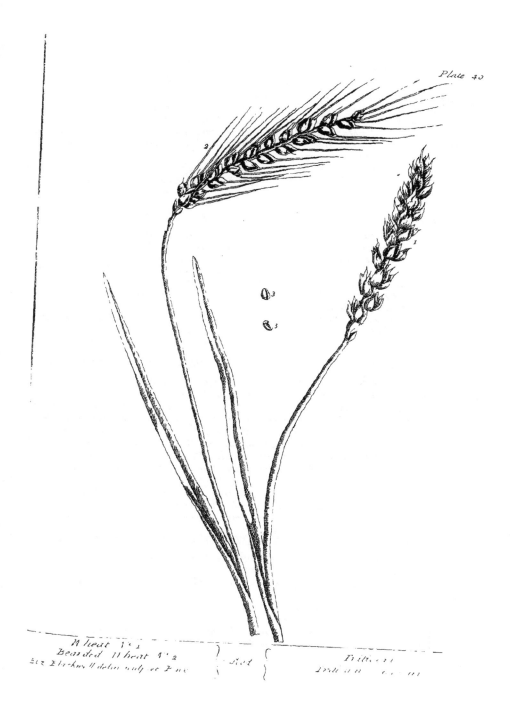

Plate 43

Wheat N.º 1
Bearded Wheat N.º 2
Eliz Blackwell delin sculp et Pinx
Tritici
Triticum

Plate 41 Verveir Verbena & Verbenaca

It grows to be two Foot high, the Stalks are a purplish Brown, the Leaves a willow Green and the Flowers pale Purple
1 It grows in Highways, near Towns & Villages, flowring in July
3 The Whole Herb is used being accounted cephalic, good against Diseases, arising from Cold and phlegmatic Causes Some commend it to open Obstructions of the Liver and Spleen, help the Jaundice and Gout Outwardly it is esteem'd vulnerary, good for sore watery inflamed Eyes
4 Greek, Περιστερεών Latin, Verbenaca supina Spanish, Berbena Italian. Verminacola French. Vervaine masse German, Eisencraut Dutch Yserkruyd

---

Plate 42 Ox-Eye-Daisy, the Great Daisy Bellis major

1 The Stalks grow more than a Foot high, the Leaves are a deep grass Green, & the Flowers white with a yellow Thrum in the middle
2 It grows in Pasture Grounds, and flowers in June
3 The Flowers of this Daisy are esteem'd balsamic good for all Disorders of the Breast and Lungs, as coughs shortness of Breath, Pleurisies, Consumptions and Wasting of the Flesh They are frequently put into Apozems and Decoctions for inward Bruises, Wounds, and Ruptures
4 Greek Βόφθαλμον Latin, Bellis major Spanish, Buphthalmo Italian. Occhio di Bue French. Oiel de Beuf German Rinds Aug Dutch, Groote Maagdeheyen

---

Plate 43 Pimpernel or Male Pimpernel Anagallis terrestris mas

1 It grows to be a Foot high, the Leaves are a grass Green and the Flowers scarlet
2 It grows in Corn Feilds flowring in May and June
3 This Plant is moderatly warm & dry with a little stipticity, and by some is accounted a good vulnerary The Juice taken inwardly, (by it self or mix'd with Cows Milk) is good in Consumptions and Distempers of the Lungs - It is often put in Cordial Waters as alexipharmic, & good against malignant Distempers Some Writers of Note have recommended it in Cases of Lunacy and Dilerious Fevers. Matthiolus commends ye Juice, for ye Tooth-Ach, snuffed up the Nostril on that Side where the Pain does not lie
4 Greek Αναγαλλίς Latin Anagallis mas Spanish Muruges Italian Anagallo French. Mouron German. Gauch heil Dutch Bastard Muur

---

Plate 44 Pansies or Hearts-Ease Viola tricolor Jaccea Flos Trinitatis

1 It grows a Foot high, the Leaves are a dark Green the Flowers spotted with a light Purple, a deep Purple and Yellow
2 It grows Wild in the Borders of Fields and is also planted in Gardens flowring great Part of the Summer
3 The Leaves are esteemed mucilaginous and vulnerary, good to take off the Gripes in Children, and prevent the Fits arising from them
4 Greek. Εστάχσουν Latin Jaccea Spanish. Yerva de S Trinadados Italian Jaccea French. Pensees German Gibenfarben Blumlin Dutch Penseen

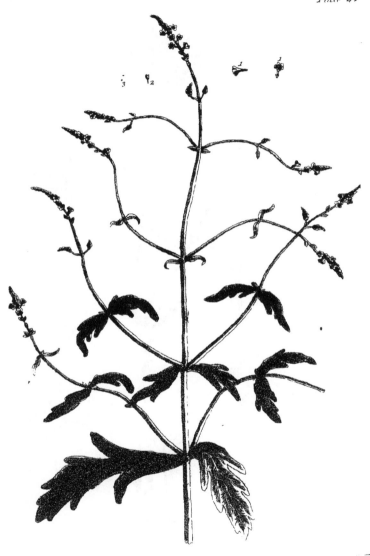

Vervain

c. Blackwell delin. sculp et Pin

1 Flower
2 a?
3 Seed

Verbena

Plate 42

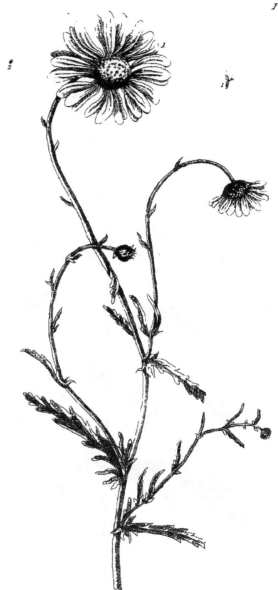

Ox Eye Daisy

Eliz Blackwell delin sculp et Pinx

} 1 Flower
} 2 Seed

Bellis major

Plate 43

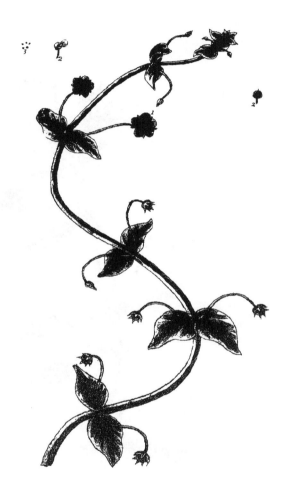

Pumpernell

Eliz. Blackwell delin sculp et Pinx

1 Flower
2 Fruit
3 Seed

Anagallis terrestris

Plate 44

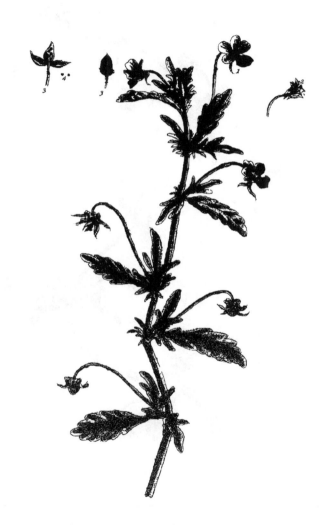

Hearts Ease
Pansies
ch. Blacknell lehm culp et Pinx

1 Flower
2 Flower by
3 Seed Vessel
4 Seed

Viola tricolor

Plate 45 Bramble or Blackberry Bush Rubus or Rubus vulgaris

1 This Shrub has many long creeping Branches, there are commonly 5 Leaves on one Footstalk in the lower Parts, and three on the upper Parts next ye Fruit the Leaves are a deep Green, the Flowers a pale Red, and sometimes White and the Fruit when ripe is of a black Colour
2 It grows in most Hedges, & flowers in Iune & Iuly the Fruit is ripe in September
3 The Leaves are accounted restringent, & are frequently prescribed in Gargarisms for sore Mouths & Throats, the unripe Fruit is very binding and restringent, useful for all kinds of Fluxes & Bleeding, for Thrushes & sore Mouths The Iuice of the ripe Fruit made into Syrup is esteemed good against the Heat of Urine
4 Greek Báros Latin. Rubus, & Rubus vulgaris Spanish Carza Italian, Rovo French, Ronce German, Briamen Brambeer and Grakbeer Dutch Braam-bezein

Plate 46 Betony Betonica, & Betonica silvestris or vulgaris

1 It grows to be eighteen Inches high the Leaves are a deep grass Green, and the Flowers a red Purple
2 Betony grows in Woods & Thickets & by Hedge sides, & flowers in May and Iune
3 It is accounted a good cephalic, hepatick & vulnerary Plant The Ancients had it so much in esteem that Antonius Musa, Physician to Augustus Caesar, wrote a whole Treatise on it The Leaves dried & mix'd with Tobacco are frequently smoaked for the Head Ach, Vertigo, & sore Eyes Mixd with Wood-Sage & Ground-Pine it makes a good diet Drink for the Gout & Rheumatism The fresh leaves bruised are good for green Wounds & to drain out Splinters The officinal preparations are the conserve of the Flowers, and the Emplastrum de Betonica
4 Greek Κεσεγν & Ψυχότροφον Latin. Betonica Spanish Bretonia Italian Betone, a French Betoine German, Betonien Dutch Betonie

Plate 47 Marum, or Syrian mastic Thyme Marum Syriacum

1 This Plant grows to be a Foot high the Leaves are willow Green, & ye Flowers red
2 It grows naturally in Candy and Syria, and is nursed up here in ye Gardens of the Curious, and flowers in Iuly
3 Marum is accounted a good cephalic and nervine Plant, and is much used in cephalic Snuff, but is of little service else in Physick
4 Greek Μάρον ή νοοβειον Latin Marum Syriacum, or Majorana and Cretica, or Marum cretense. Spanish,   Italian Maro French German   Dutch,

Plate 48 Brooklime Anagalis aquatica or Becabunga

1 It grows to be sixteen Inches high the Leaves are a grass Green, and the Stalks a reddish Green, and the Flowers a fine Blue
2 This Plant grows in Rills & running Ditches, it flowers in Iune & keeps its Leaves all ye Winter
3 It is accounted a good dealstruent & antiscorbutic abounding with volatile Parts very good for ye Scurvy being an Ingredient of ye antiscorbutic Iuices & diet Drinks for that Distemper is is likewise detersive & cleansing useful in obstructions or ye Kidneys by Gravel or slimy Humours, is this prime Stone & Dropsy Matthiolus says it is good to bring away a false conception & provoke the Menses
4 Greek Αναγαλλις, Latin Anagallis aquatica & Becabunga Spanish   Italian French Berle German Wasserbungen and Bachbunsem Dutch Bekelmn & Beck pung, n

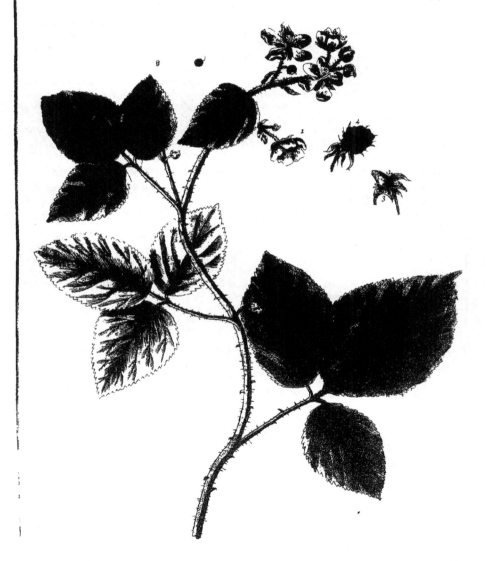

Black Berry Bush

chz Blackwell delin. sculp. et Pinx

1 Flower
2 Fruit
3 Seed Vessell

Rubus

Plate 4

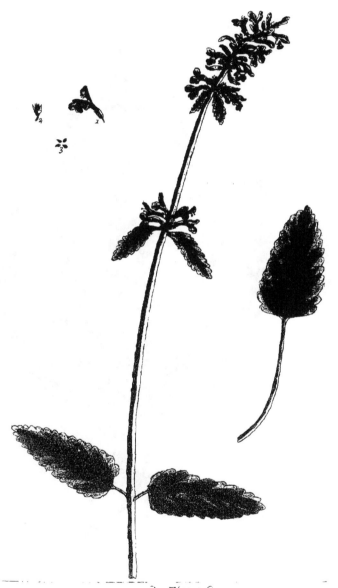

Betony

Euz Blackwell delin sculp et Pinx

{ 1 Flower
{ 2 cup
{ 3 seed

Betonica

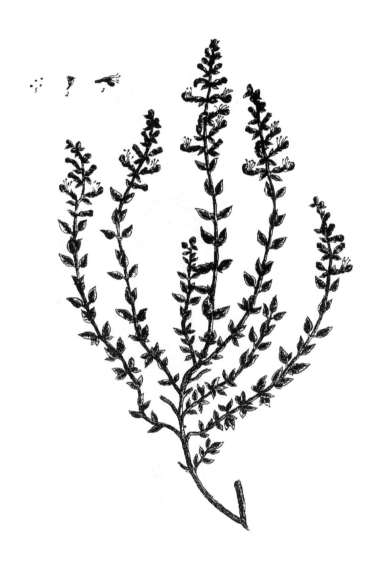

Marum

Elız Blackwell delin. sculp.

2 Flower
2 cup
Seed

Marum germanicum

Plate 48

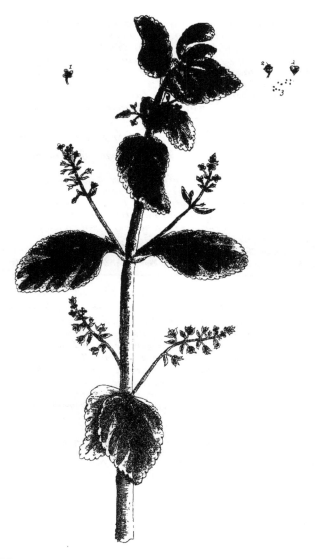

Brook Lime 　　　1 *Flower* 　　　*Anagallis aquatica*

Zaz Bachwell delin caul, a Pinx 　2 *Seed Vessell* 　*Beerlumer*
　　　　　　　　　　　　　　3 *Seet*

Plate 49 *Spinge Spinachia*

1. It grows to be two Foot high, the Leaves are a grass Green and the Flowers a light yellowish Green

2. It is sown yearly in Gardens, and flowers according to the Month it is sown in

3. Spinage is more used for Food than Medicine, being a good boild Sallad, and much eaten in the Spring, as good to temper the Heat & Sharpness of the Humours it is esteemed cooling, moistning, & diuretic. rendring the Body soluble Serapius an Arabian Physician says, that Spinage creates Wind, so that those who are troubled Chollic had better not eat it

4. Greek Σπαναχιον Latin, Spinachia or Lapathum hortense. Spanish Spanache Italian, Spinache French, Espinoches German. Spinat Dutch Spinacie

---

Plate 50 *Wild Teasel Dipsacus silvestris or Labrum veneris*

1. This Teasel grows to be four or five Foot high. the Leaves are a light grass green, and the Flowers purple

2. It grows upon Banks in the borders of Fields, and flowers in June and July

3. The Roots are esteemed cleansing the Antients commend a Decoction of them in Wine, boiled to a Consistence & kept in a brazen Vessel to be applied to ij Rhagades, or Clests of the Fundament and for a Fistula therein, and to take away Warts The Water found in the hollow of the Leaves is commended as a Collyrium to cool Inflammations of the Eyes, and as a Cosmetic to render the Face fair

4. Greek Δίψακος Latin Dipsacus silvestris or Labrum veneris Spanish Cardencha or Cardo penteador Italian, Cardo da Panni & Dissaco French. Cardon German. dissel Dutch. Groote Wildekaarden

---

Plate 51 *Pilewort or small Celendine Chelidonium minus*

1. The Stalks grow to be 6 or 8 Inches high, the Leaves are a dark Green, and the Flowers a fine bright Yellow, the Root resembles the Piles in the Human Body

2. It grows in Meadows & moist Pastures, & by Hedges, and flowers in March & April

3. This Herb is accounted to be good for the Haemorrhoides or Piles, to ease their Pain and Swelling & stop their bleeding the Roots being taken inwardly & an Ointment made of the Leaves & Roots applied outwardly Some commend it for the Jaundice & Scurvy especially in the Mouth, to strengthen the Gums and preserve the Teeth

· Greek Κελιδόνιον μικρόν Latin. Chelidonium minus Spanish Scrofolaria menor Italian Chelidonia minore French. Coulos de Prestres German. Pfaffenhödlin Dutch. Kelynspeen kruyt

---

Plate 52 *Primrose Primula Veris*

The Stalks grow to be eight or ten Inches high the Leaves are a grass Green & the Flowers a pale Yellow, and the Roots a reddish Purple

It grows in Thickets and under Hedges and flowers in March and April.

The Flowers are commended as good against Disorders arising from phlegmatic Humours The Juice of the Root is used as an Errhine to purge the Head of tough slimy Phlegm

Greek   Latin Primula Veris Spanish   Italian Fiore di Primo vera French. Primevere German. Schlüssellblumen Dutch Groote Wilde sleutel blom

Plate 49

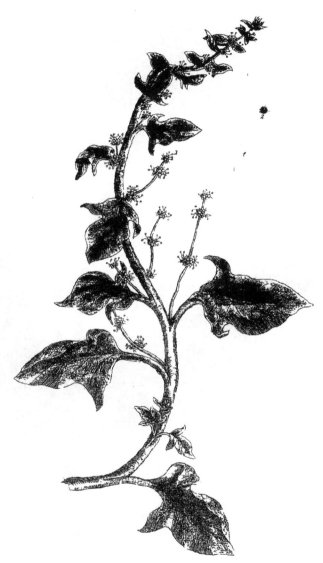

Spinage

{ 1 Flower
{ 2 Seed

Spinachia

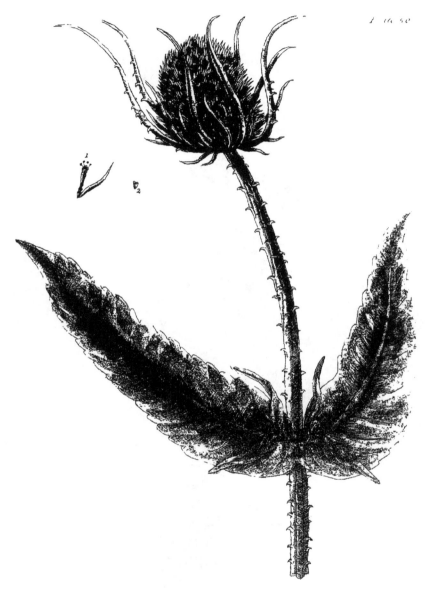

t. 80

1

2

Wild Teasel
Herbal Vol. III. tab. 102

{ 1 Flower
{ 2 Seed

Dipsacus silvestris
Libium I.

Plate 51

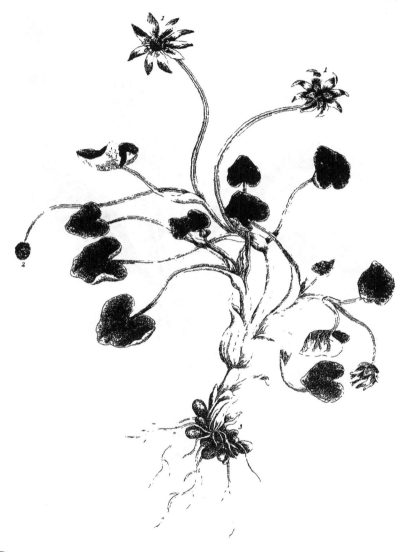

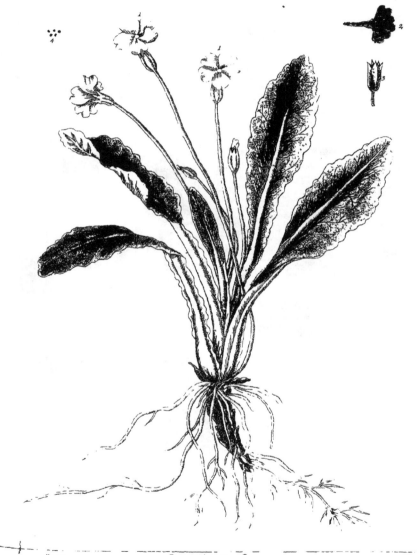

Plate 52

Primrose

lthe Blossid the other Pimn

1 Flower
2 Separate Flower
3 cup
4 seed

Primula veris

Plate 53 *Male Satyrion, or Male Fools-Stones. Satyrium mas*

1. This Orchis, which is the common Satyrion of the Shops, grows to be a Foot high, the Leaves are a bright Green spotted with Black, and the Flowers, which grow on a brownish Stalk, are a Red Purple.
2. It grows in moist Meadows, and flowers in April and May.
3. The Roots are accounted a Stimulus to Venery, strengthening the Genital Parts, and helping Conception, and for these Purposes are a chief Ingredient in the Electuarium Diasatyrium.
   Outwardly they are applied in form of a Cataplasm, and are esteemed good to dissolve hard Tumours and Swellings.
   The Officinal Preparation is the Electuarium Diasatyrum.
   Dioscorides says, that the Roots of this Plant boiled and eat by Men makes them beget Boys, and the Roots of the Female Satyrion eat by Women makes them Conceive Girls.
4. Greek, ὄρχις Theophrastus Σατύριον ὀρχιῶδες, Dioscorides Latin, Satyrium mas or Testiculus morionis Spanish, Coyon de perro Italian Testacolo di Cane French, Couillon de Prestres German, Schmal Knabencraut meunle Dutch, Kulleyes kruyd.

Plate 54 *Hollyhorks. Malva hortensis*

1. This Plant grows six or seven Foot high, the Leaves are a light green, and the Flowers a pale Red.
2. It grows in Gardens, and flowers in July and August.
3. Hollyhocks are much of the Nature of the common Mallows vid Plate 22 but less mollifying, they are mostly used in Gargles, for the Swelling of the Tonsils, and Relaxation of the Uvula.
4. Greek ἡμέρα μαλάχη. Camerarius Latin., Malva hortensis Spanish Malvas Italian. Malva maggiore French. Malves de Jardin German. Ernrosen Dutch, Stockroosen.

Plate 55 *March Violet. Viola martia.*

1. The Stalks of this Violet creep on the Ground, the Leaves are a dark Green and the Flowers a blue Purple.
2. It grows wild in Hedges and is cultivated when used in Gardens, and flowers in March.
3. The Flowers are one of the four Cordial Flowers, & esteemed cooling, moystning and laxative, good in Affections of the Breast and Lungs, helping Coughs and pleuretic Pains.
   The Syrup is given to Children to open and cool their Bodies.
   The Leaves are cooling and opening and frequently put into Glisters and Ointments against Inflammations.
   The Seed is reckon'd good for the Stone and Gravel.
   The Officinal Preparation is the Syrupus Violarum.
4. Greek ἰόλα λου. Dioscorides Latin Viola martia Spanish, Violetta Italian Viola French. Violette German Merken Biolen Dutch, Diole.

Plate 56 *White Saxifrage Saxifraga alba*

1. White Saxifrage grows to be a foot high, the Leaves are a light Green and the Flowers White, with yellow Apices.
2. It grows in Meadows and flowers in April and May.
3. This Plant takes its Name from its supposed Virtues being diuretic and lithontriptic good for the Stone and Gravel, and Stoppage of Urine.
   The Officinal Preparation is the Simple Water.
4. Greek
   French   Latin Saxifraga alba Spanish   Italian
                 German   Dutch Steenbreuk

Plate 53

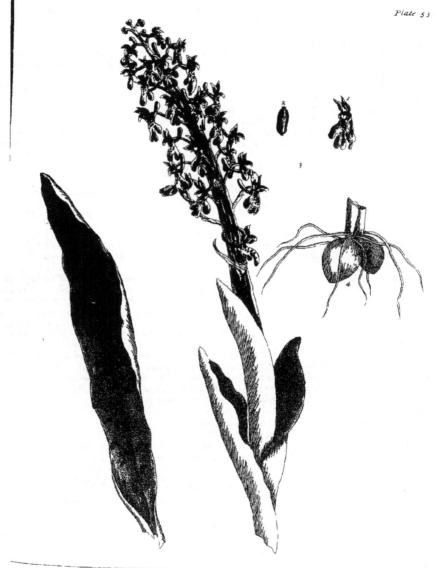

Male Satyrion

Enz Black's ell I lin sculp et Pinx

1 Flower
2 Fruit
3 Leaf
4 Root

Satyrium mas

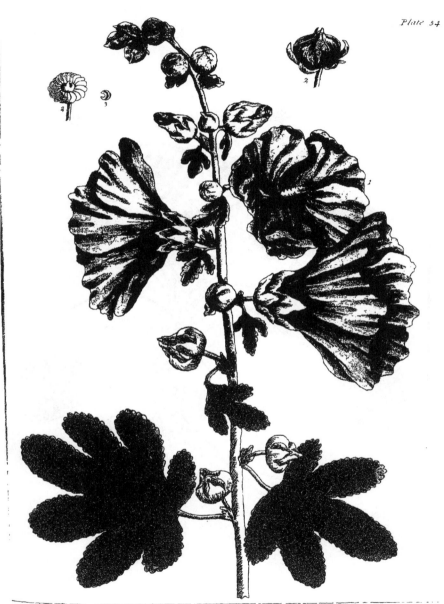

Plate 54

Hollyhocks

1 Flower

2 Fruit

3 red

Malua arborea

Euz Blackwell delin sulp et Pinx

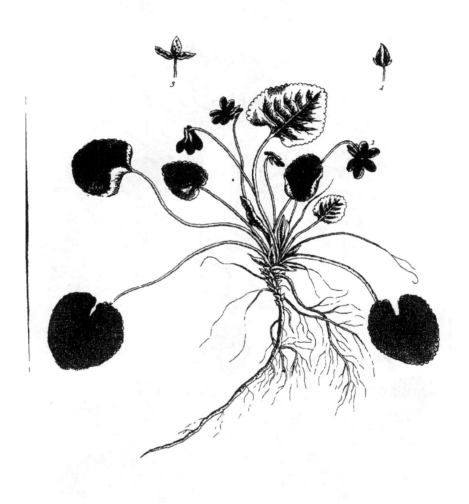

March Violet

Eliz Blackwell delin. sculp et Pinx

1 Flower
2 Fruit
3 Seed Vessell & c

Viola Martia

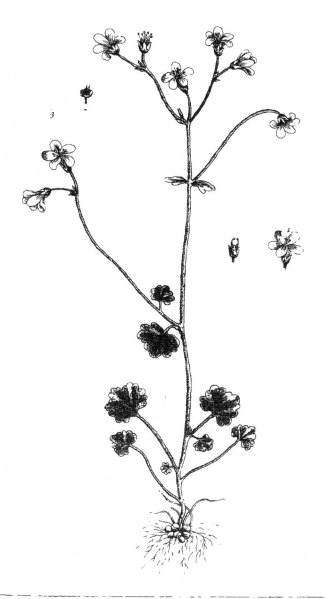

White Saxifrage

Eliz. Blackwell del. sculp et Pinx

1 Flowers
2 Fruit
3 Seed

Saxifraga alba

Plate 57 Bears-foot, or Black Hellebore Helleborastes

1 It grows to be 18 Inches high, the Bottom Leaves are dark Green, and the upper light green, the Flowers are a very light Green tinctured with Purple round the Edges

2 It grows on the Mountains of Swiserland, Austria, and Susia, and is planted with us in Gardens, and Flowers the latter end of December, whence it is called the Christmass Flower

3 Bears-foot was esteemed by the Ancients good for Melancholy and Madness to purge black choler and Humours ariseing thence, they likewise gave it in Jeprosies, Shingles, the Itch and the like Cutaneous Affections It is also commended for the Gout, and of late it has been very much made use of in stubborn Obstructions of the Catamenia The officinal Medicine is the Tinctura Ellebori

4 Greek, Ελλέβοεος μέλας Dioscorides Latin, Elleborum nigrum, or Helleborus, ier Spanish Verde gambre nero, or Elleboro Italian, Elleboro nero French Ellebore noire German, Christwurt Dutch

---

Plate 58 Doves-foot, or Crane's Bill Geranium Columbinum or Pes columbinus

1 This Species of Cranes Bill grows a foot high the Leaves at the Bottom spread on the Ground, and are a bright Green the stalks are a Reddish Green, and the Flowers a red Purple

2 It grows on Banks and Flowers great Part of the Summer

3 It is esteemed a vulnerary Plant, usefull in inward Wounds Bruises and Haemorrhagies and all Fluxes It is much cry'd up for the Cure of Ruptures in Children given in Pouder It also helps the stone and provokes Urine

4 greek, Γεεάνιον Dioscorides Latin, Geranium columbinum Spanish Pico de Cinquenha Italian Geranio French, Bec de Cicongue German, Belscher Storchschnabel Dutch, Duyvevoet

---

Plate 59 Periwinckle, Vinca pervinca, or Clematis Daphnoides

1 Periwinckle grows a foot high, the Leaves are a bright shineing Green and the Flowers a blew Purple but sometimes white

2 It grows in shady Banks & dry Ditches, & Flowers most Months in ye Summer

3 It is accounted a good vulnerary Plant, & is often used in Wound-Drinks for Bruises, Contusions, inward Bleeding, Wasting & spitting of Blood & ye Excess of ye Catamenia & ye Fluor albus

4 greek, Κλήματις δαφνοίδης Dioscorides Latin, Vinca pervinca Spanish Pervinqua, Italian, Provenca French, Lyserum German Singrun Dutch, Vincoorde

---

Plate 60 Wood-roof Asperula odorata, or Aspergula

1 The Stalks grow to be a foot high, ye Leaves are a deep grass Green, & ye Flowers white

2 It grows in Woods and Copses, and Flowers in May

3 Wood roof is esteemed a good Hepatic and usefull against Inflammations of the Liver Obstructions of the Gall Bladder, and Jaundise The Germans put it into their Wine as we do Borrage & Burnet, as a great Cordial and Comforter of the Spirits The Green Herb bruised is applyed by ye Countrey Folks to hot Tumours, Inflammations and fresh Cuts

4 greek Λευκεόδαρον ασερον Dioscorides Latin Asperula odorata Spanish Rubia Italian Rubia salvatica French garence german Bildt Rot Dutch

16 15

Plate 5.

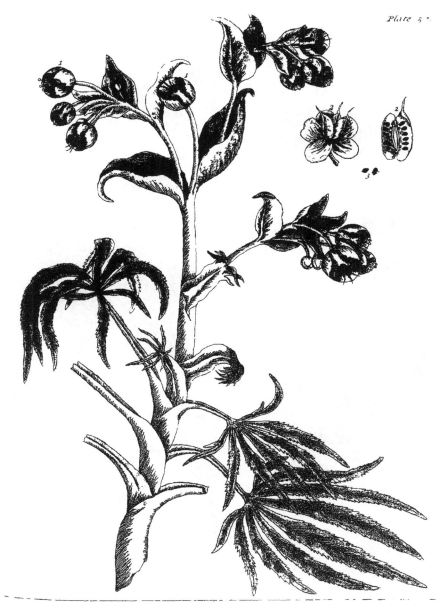

Bears foot

Elix. Blackwell delin. sculp et pinx.

1 Flores
2 Pods Pods pin
3 seed

Telleboraster

Plate 53.

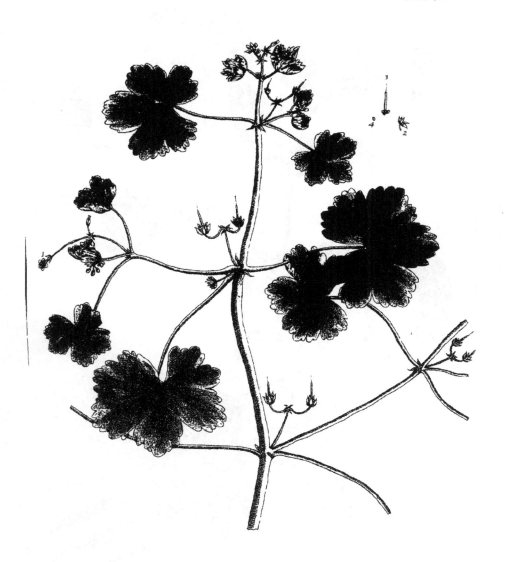

Dove's foot
Crane's Bill

1. Flower
2. cup
3. seed vessel
4. seed

Geranium columbinum
Pe columbinu

Eliz Blackwell delin sculp et Pinx

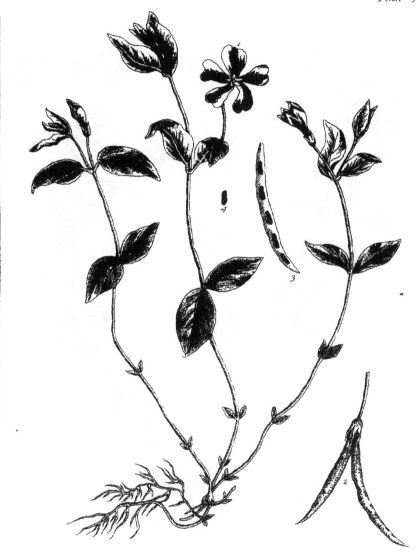

Plate 59

Periwinkle

Vinca Pervinca
Diphneides

Plate 90

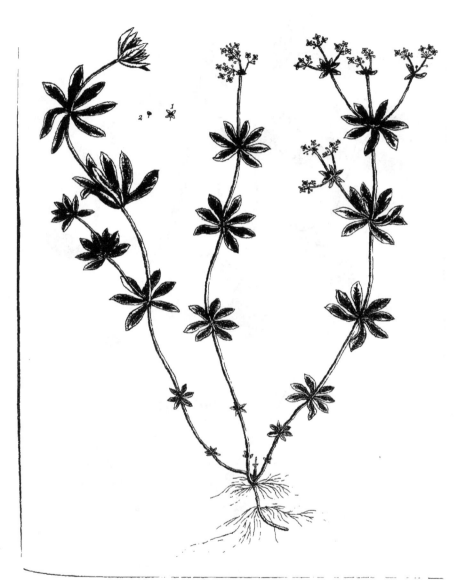

Wood 1005

Mrs Blackwell delin sculp et pinx

1 Flower

2 Seed

Asperula odorata

Asperula

Plate 61. Hyacinth or Hare-bells Hyacinthus

1. The Stalk grows 8 or 9 Inches high, the Leaves are a grass Green, the Flowers commonly a deep blew, but sometimes flesh colour and sometimes white
2. It grows in Hedges and Woods, and Flowers in May
3. The Roots are used, and esteemed by some diuretic, and good to stop all kinds of Fluxes
4. Greek Ὑάκινθος   Latin, Hyacinthus Spanish, Maros flores Italian Hyacintho French, Vacciet or Jacinte german Merkenblumen Dutch Hyacinthe

Plate 62 Spurge Laurel Laureola

1. This Shrub grows 3 foot high, the Leaves are a dark Green, and the Flowers a yellow Green
2. It grows in Woods and Thickets, and Flowers in March and April, and the Fruit is ripe in September
3. The Leaves and Berries are used by some, as good to purge Bile choleric and serous Humours, but they purge with great Violence both upwards and downwards Some Adventurous Persons give them in Dropsies
4. Greek Δαφνοειδἑς   Latin Laureola Spanish   Italian. Laureola French. Laureole german Cross Kellershalfs Dutch

Plate 63 Sanicle or Self-Heal Sanicula or Diapentia

The Stalks grow to be a Foot high the Leaves are a bright grass Green, and the Flowers white
2. It grows in Woods and Flowers in May
3. This is one of the Chief vulnerary Plants being frequently put into Wound-Drinks and traumatic Apozems, and is esteemed good for Ruptures inward Bruises spitting of Blood, or any Haemorrhages, and Wounds both inward and outward
4. Greek   Latin Sanicula or Diapentia spanish Italian, Cinquefoglia Maggiore French. La Sanicle german Sanidel Dutch

Plate 64 Bugle or middle Confound Bugula, or Consolida media

The Stalks on which the Flowers grow are 9 Inches high the Leaves are a Reddish Green, and the Flowers a bright Blue
2. It grows in Woods and Hedges, and Flowers in May
3. Bugle is a noted vulnerary Plant and used inwardly & outwardly for all kinds of Bruises, Wounds and Contusions as likewise for Sores Ulcers Spitting of Blood and Hamorrhagies from any Part
4. Greek   Latin Bugula or Consolida media spanish Italian   french Bugle german Gulden guntel Dutch

Plate 65

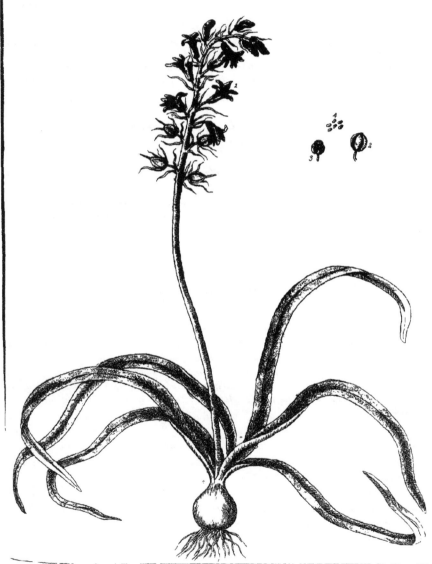

1 Flower
2 Seed Vessell
3 Seed Vessell open
4 Seed

Hyacinthus.

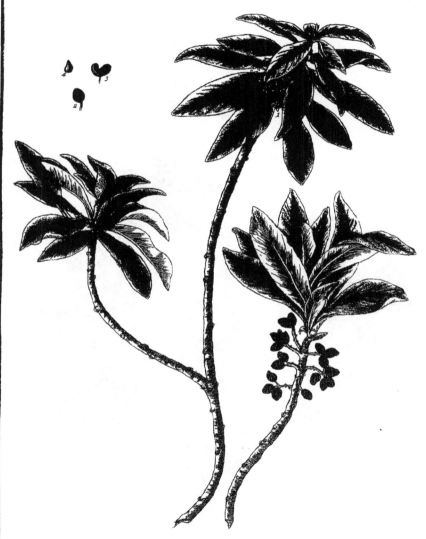

Plate [illegible]

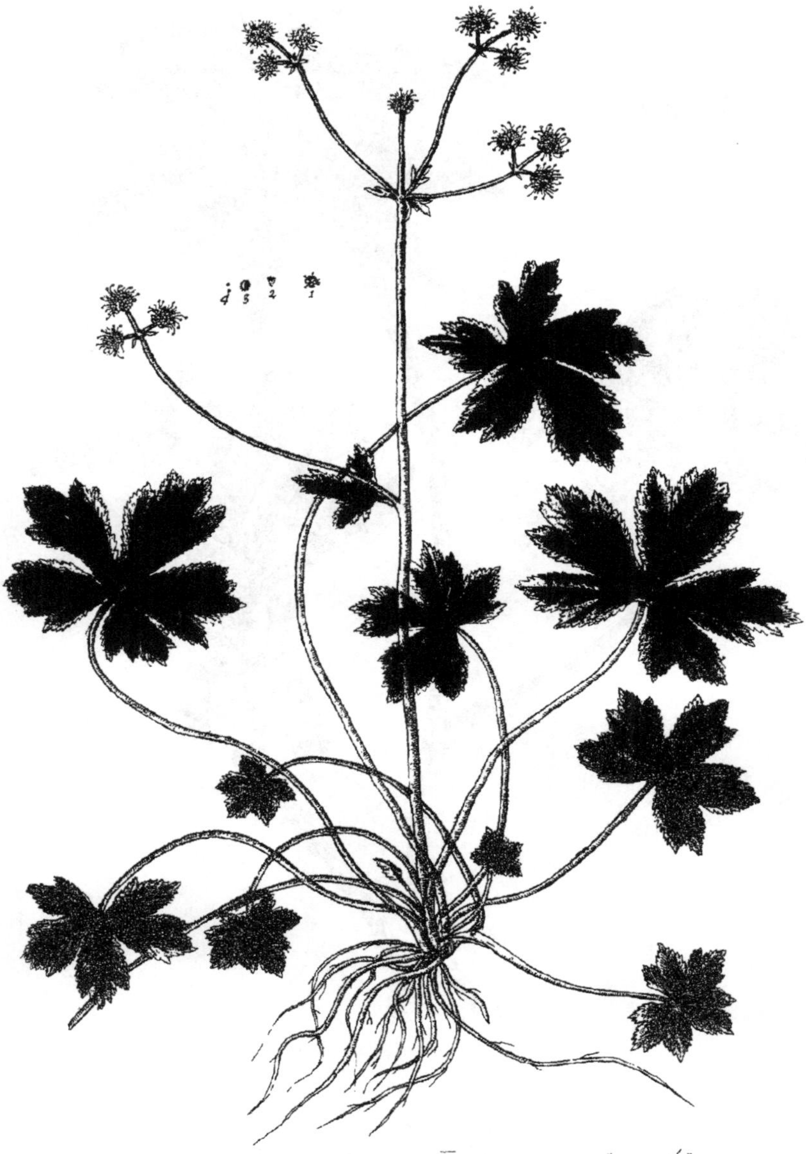

Sanicle
[illegible] heal
[illegible] et Pinx

1 Flower
2 Calix
3 Seed Vessell
4 Seed

Sanicula
Diapensia

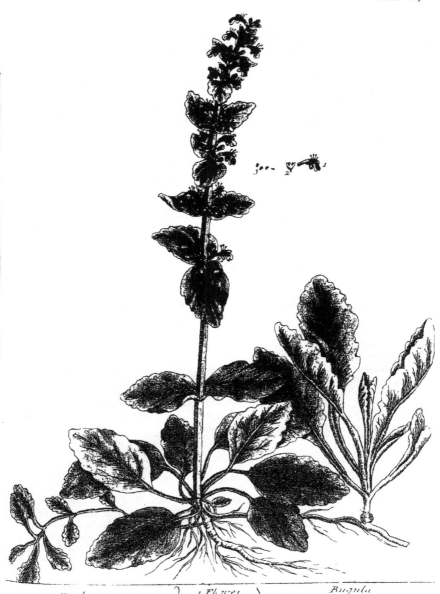

Bugula

Plate 65 The *Female Piony* Paeonia faemina

1 It grows 2 or 3 foot high ye Leaves are a grass Green & the Flowers a fine Crimson

2 It is cultivated in Gardens, and *flowers in April and May*

3 This Plant generally Supplies the Place of ye Male Piony, and is accounted good for the Epilepsy, Apoplexy and all kinds of Convulsions and nervous Affections, both in young & old Some recommend it in histeric Cases the Obstructions of ye Menses, and ye Retention of the *Lochia* The Root and Seed are hung about Childrens Necks to prevent Convulsions in breeding their Teeth

4 Greek, Γλυκυσίδη or Παιονία Θηλεία Latin Paeonia faemina Spanish Rosa del monte or Rosa albardeira Italian Peonia French, Pivoine or Pynoine German Peonien Dutch

---

Plate 66 The great *Blew-bottle* Cyanus major

1 It grows 10 Inches high the Leaves are a deep Green on the Inside and a light Green on the Backside, the Flowers are a full blue

2 It grows in Gardens and *Flowers in Iune*

3 This is reckoned among the vulnerary Plants, the Iuice being commended against Bruises and Contusions which come of Falls though a Vein be broken and the Party spit Blood, as also to heal any Cut or green Wound

4 Greek, Κύανος Latin, Cyanus major Spanish, Italian Fior Campese, fior Aliso, & Battifuocero French German Cornblum Dutch Groote blommen

---

Plate 67 *May-Weed, or faetid Camomile* cotula faetida

1 It grows about a foot high the Leaves are a dark Green and the Flowers white with a yellow Thrum in the middle

2 It grows amongst the Corn and on Banks, and waste Places and *Flowers for* several Months in the Summer

3 Some Authours commend this Plant as good against Vapours and Hysteric Fits Mr Ray says, It was sometimes used in Scrophulous Cases Tournefort says That about Paris they use it in Fomentations for Pains and Swellings of Haemorrhuges

4 Greek Ἄνθεμις and Ἄνθεμον Latin Cotula faetida & Chamaemelum faetidum Spanish Manzanilla Italian, Camamilla French Camenima or Camomille German Camillen Dutch Stinkende Camille

---

Plate 68 *Treacle Mustard* Thlaspi

1 This Plant grows to be a foot high the Leaves are a grass Green and the Flowers are white

2 It grows in Corn-fields in Essex and *Flowers in May*

3 It is hot and dry and somewhat diuretic, and is esteemed good to provoke Urine and to help the Dropsy Gout Sciatica and forward the Menstrual Evacuations The Seed of this Plant is what ought to be used in the Theriaca & Mithridate but being scarcely to be had the Seed of the Mithridate Mustard or Thlaspi vulgatissimum may be used as a Succedaneum for it

4 Greek Θλάσπι Latin, Thlaspi Spanish Paniqueso de flor blanco Italian Thlaspi French Seneve Saurage German Besenkraut Dutch Boeren kersse

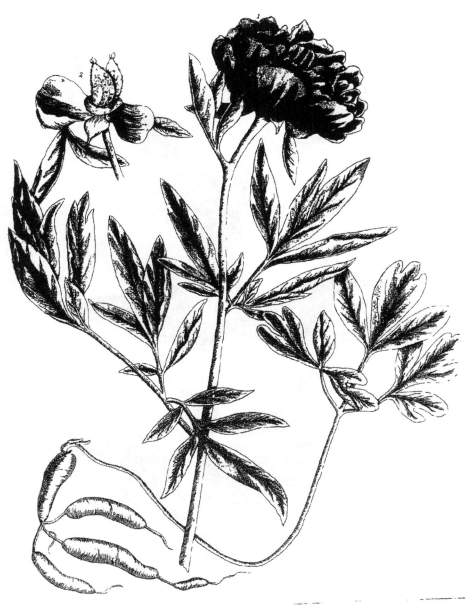

Plate 5

Female Pæony

$\left\{\begin{array}{l}\text{1 Flower}\\\text{2 Seed Vessel}\end{array}\right.$

Pæonia fæmina

Eliz Blackwell delin. sculp. et Pinx.

Plate 60.

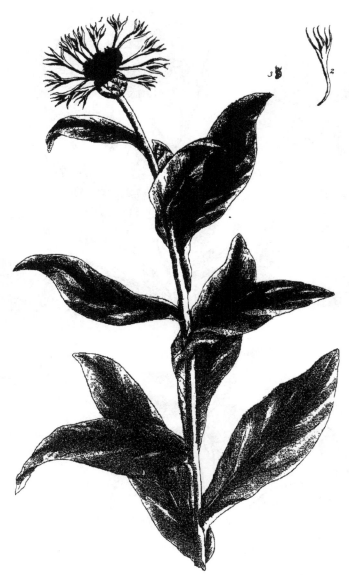

The great Blew-bottle

t 12 Blackwell delin. sculp et Pinx.

1 Flower
2 Flower aperta
3 Seed

Cyanus maior

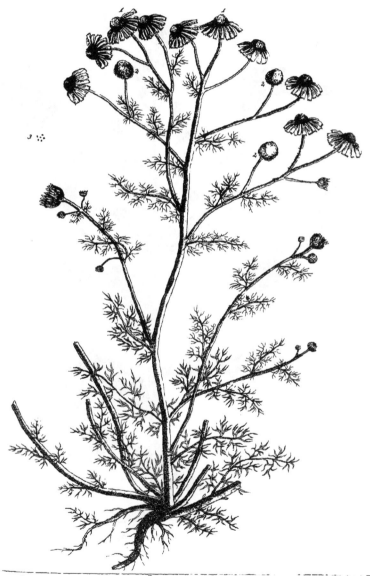

May Weed ɳ Field Camomile   1 Fl ner   *Chamæmelum vulgare*
Vlit Blackwell delin ch et Pinx   2 Fruit

Plate 98

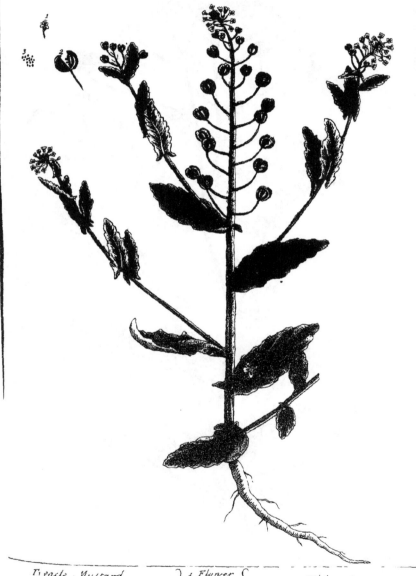

Treacle Mustard

Eliz Blackwell delin sculp et Pinx

1 Flower
2 Seed Vessel
3 Seed

Thlaspi

Plate 69 *Garden Flower de-luce* Iris nostras hortensis

1 It grows to be 18 Inches high, the Leaves are a light Green, & ỹ Flowers a bluish Purple
2 It grows in Gardens, and Flowers in May
3 The Juce of the Root is a strong Errhine, when snuff'd up the Nostrils it purges ỹ Head and clears the Brain of thin serous phlegmatic Humors
  a strong Decoction of the Root given inwardly is a strong Vomit and accounted good for the Dropsy, Jaundice and Ague
  This Vomit is very offensive to the Stomach
4 Greek I'eis   Latin Iris nostras hortensis Spanish, Lirio Cardeno Italian Giglio celeste French Flambe German, Blau gilgen Beilwart Dutch, Lisch

---

Plate 70 *Lillies of the Valley* Lilium convallium

1 It grows to be 8 or 10 Inches high, the Leaves are a grass green and the Flowers white
2 It grows in the Vallies, but chiefly in Gardens, and flowers in May and June
3 Lillies of the Valley are of great service in all Disorders of the Head and Nerves as Apoplexy Epilepsy, Palsy, Convulsions Vertigo
  They are much used in Errhines and cephalic Snuff
  a Large quantity of them are put in the Aqua Paeoniae C and spirit Lavendular C and the Aq Antepileptica
4 Greek   Latin, Lilium convallium Spanish
  Italian Lilia convallis French, Muguat german, Reyenblumlin Dutch Lelie-van den Daalen

This Insea was travelling upon the Lilly but it feeds commonly upon fruit Trees & is called ỹ Tuckey from its variety of Colours

---

Plate 71 *Sage of Vertue* Salvia minor or virtutis

1 The stalks grow to be 18 Inches high ỹ Leaves are a light green and ỹ Flowers a pale Purple
2 It grows in Gardens and flowers in May and June
3 It is esteem'd good for all Diseases of the Head and Nerves as ỹ Palsy Convulsions &c They use it likewise for Uterine obstructions, and in Fevers of all sorts
  The Leaves are used in the Aq Antepileptica Antiparalytica Titne Composita Syrup Stoechados Ung Masatum Caspar Commelin
4 Greek Σφάκελος Latin, Salvia minor, or Salvia virtutis Spanish Salvia or Salvia menore Italian Salvia minore French   German
       Dutch, Salie

Plate 72 *Ladie's mantle* Alchimilla

1 It grows to be a foot high the Leaves are a grass Green and ỹ Flowers a yellow green
2 It grows in Meadow and Pasture Grounds, and flowers in May
3 This Plant is reckn'd a good vulnerary, being drying & binding incrassating and consolidating and of great force to stop inward Bleeding the immoderate Flux of the Menses and the Fluor albus
  The Leaves applyed outwardly are accounted good for lank flaggong Breasts to bring them to a greater Fumness and smaller Compass
4 Green,   Latin Alchimilla Spanish
  Italian Stellaria French Pie de Lyon German Synnau   Dutch Synnau onser Drouven mantel

N 18

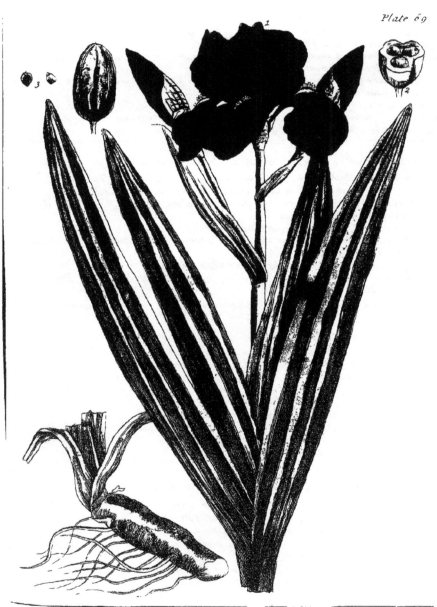

Plate 69

Garden Flower-de-Luce

Eliz Blackwell delin sculp et Pinx

1. Flower
2. Seed Vessell
3. Seed

Iris Jermax hortensis

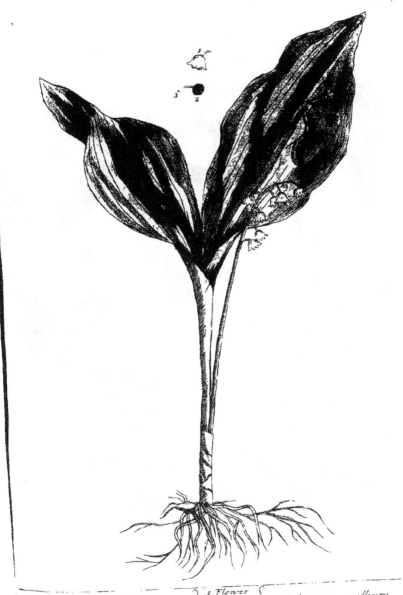

Plate 70

Lillies of the Valley   Lilium convallium

Eliz Blackwell delin sulp et Pinx   1 Flower
                                     2 Berry
                                     3 Seed
                                     4 the Leaf. 4

Plate *1

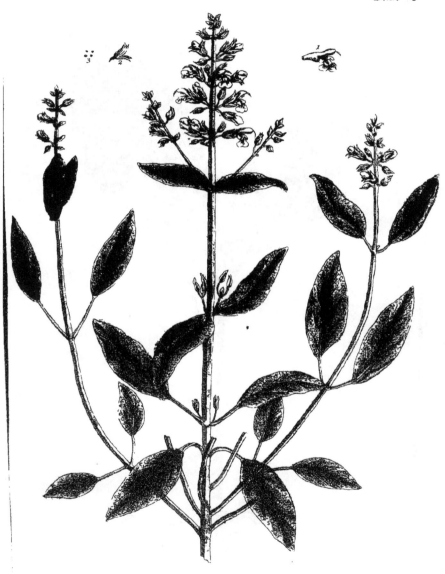

Sage of Vertue
Eliz: Blackwell delin: sculp: et Pinx

1 Flower
2 Seed vessell
3 Seed

Salvia minor
Salvia nostras

Plate 7 ª

2 ⅓ *1*

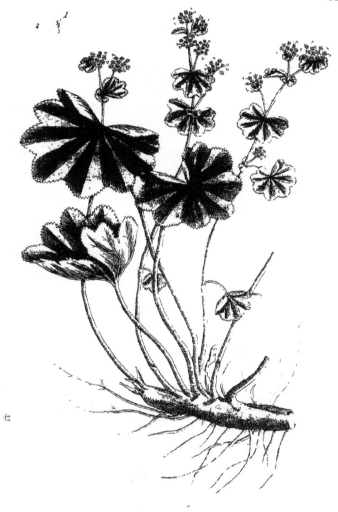

Ladies Mantle   } 1 Flower {   Alchimilla
Eliz Blackwell del'n sculp et Pinx } 2 Seed {

Plate 73 The White Rose   Rosa alba

This Tree grows taller than most other kinds of Roses having fewer Prickles on y Branches
and those pretty large the Leaves are a dark Green, and the Flowers white
It grows in Gardens, and flowers in June
The Flowers are esteemed drying, binding and cooling
The Water distilled from them is much used in Collyriums for sore inflam'd Eyes
The Officinal Preparation is the Distilled Water
Greek Ροδον λευκη   Latin Rosa alba Spanish Rosas blancos Italian Rosa bianca
French, Roses   German, Rosen Dutch Witte Roos

Plate 74 White Hellebore   Elleborum or Veratrum album

The Stalks grow to be 2, or 3 foot high , the Leaves are a bright green and the Flowers
a dull Green, or a dark Purple
It grows in the mountainous Parts of Swiserland, Austria and Stiria, with us it is
planted in Gardens, and flowers in June
The Roots are a strong Cathartic and purges with great Violence for which reason it
is but seldom given inwardly
The Powder of the Roots cause violent sneezing when snuffed up the Nostrils, and is
rarely used without milder Ingredients
This Plant outwardly applyed, is of great service in all Distempers of the Skin,   as
Tetters Scabs, Itch &c
The Officinal Preparation is the Electuarium ex Hellebore
Greek ελλεβορος λευκος Latin Elleborum album Spanish Verde gandre blanco Italian
Elleboro bianco French Verare or Ellebore blanc German, Weiß Nießwurz Dutch Witte Niesswortel

---

Plate 75 White Dittany or Fraxinella   Dictamnus albus or Fraxinella

It grows to be 2 foot high the Leaves are a dark Green and y Flowers red & sometimes white
It grows wild in several Places of France & germany, but is planted here in Gardens & flowers in June & July
The Roots are esteemed cordial and cephalic good to resist Putrefaction and Poison and useful in
malignant and pestilental Distempers
It is accounted good for Epilepsies & other Disorders of y Head, Opening Obstructions of y Womb & procuring y Menses
The Preparations are the Aq. Antepileptic Theriacal Pulv. Liberans Empl Saptuam Paracels
Greek Χαμαιρις η δικταμον Latin Dictamnus albus, or Fraxinella Spanish Dittamo blanc
Italian Dittamo bianco French Dyptam basturde German, Gemeiner Diptam Dutch Fraxinella

---

Plate 76 Cross-wort   Cruciata

It grows to be a foot high, the Leaves are a light green, and y flowers Yellow
It grows in Hedges and the Borders of Fields, but is rarely to be met with about London
except in Mr Brooks Grounds at Hampstead it grew formerly in great plenty in Hamp
stead Church yard but they have dug it up It flowers in June
It is reckoned among the vulnerary Plants, being of a drying & binding Nature & is inwardly
commended for y swelling of y Scrotum, mst is caused by y falling down of the Intestines into it
Greek Hadrianus Junius Latin Cruciata Spanish   Italian
     French,   German   Dutch
This Caterpillar is called by some the Leopard and produces a very beautiful Moth
          see Albin History Plate 30.
No

Plate 7

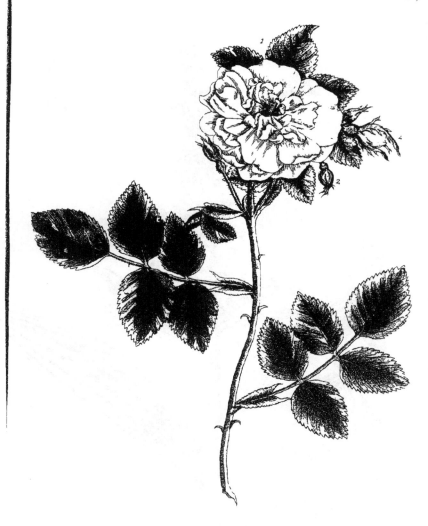

The White Rose.

M. Blackwell delin. sculp. et Pinx.

1 Flower
2 Bud

Rosa alba

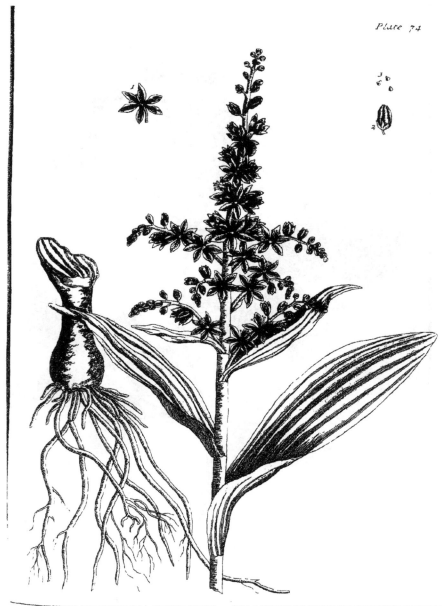

Plate 74

White Hellebore.

Eliz Blackwell di hin sculp et Pinx

{ 1 Flower
  2 Fruit
  3 Seed }

Elleborum, or Veratrum album

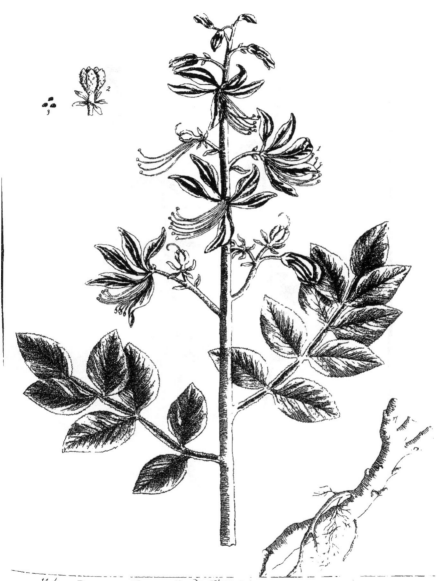

White Dittany or Fraxinella {1 Flower}
{2 Fruit}
{3 Seed}

Dictamnus albus et Fraxinella

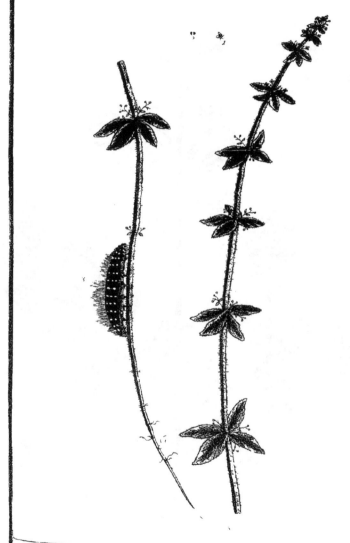

Dost nert

Eliz. Blackwell deen culp et Pinx

1. Flower
2. Seed

orientala.

Plate 77 *Strawberries Fragaria*

1. This Plant creeps upon the Ground, the Stalks on which the Fruit grows are about Eight Inches long the Leaves are a dark Grass Green, and the Flowers white

2. They grow in woods and flower in May and the Fruit is ripe in June

3. The Leaves are used in Lotions and Gargarisms for sore Mouths and Throats and Ulcers in the Gums. Some Authors commend them for the Jaundice and all kind of Fluxes.
The Fruit is accounted Cordial and good for hot bilious Constitutions, and grateful to the Stomach especially eaten with Wine and Sugar The flowers make the Aq Antinephritica. Caspar Comelin

4. Greek.   Latin. Fragaria Spanish.   Italian
Fragolaria French. Fraisier German. Bergerdbeer Dutch. Hardbesien

Plate 78 *The Red Rose. Rosa Rubra*

1. This Rose Bush is less than the white or Damask, the flowers have very few Prickles on the stalks the Leaves are a grass Green and the Flowers a light Crimson

2. It grows in Gardens and flowers in June and July

3. The Red Rose is more binding and restringent than any of the Other species x are esteemed good in all kinds of Fluxes They strengthen the Stomach prevent Vomiting stop tickling Coughs by preventing the Defluxion of Rheum and are of great Service in Consumptions The Apices are also accounted cordial
The Officinal Preparations are a Simple Water the Conserva Rosarum Sacharum Rosarum Syrupus e Rosis succis Mel Rosarum Ol Rosarum, Unguentum Rosarum Tinctura Rosarum et species Aromaticum Rosarum
Greek Pod'ov Latin Rosa rubra Spanish Rosas Italian Rosa French Roses German Rosen Dutch, Kard Rosen

Plate 79 *Ladies Thistle Carduus Mariæ*

1. The Stalks grow to be 4 or 5 foot high, the Leaves are a willow green spotted n° white, and the flowers Purple

2. It grows frequently upon Banks and Borders of fields and flowers in June

3. This Thistle is esteem'd to partake of the Virtues of y Carduus benedictus, but in a low Degree Some commend it as a Specific for the Pleurisy, especially an Emulsion of the Seeds
It is helpful also for the Jaundice, the Stone, and stoppage of Urine

4. Greek   Latin Carduus Mariae Spanish   Italian
Cardi del latte French Chardon de nostre Dame German Unser Frauen Distel.
Dutch, Onse Drauwe Distel

Plate 80 *Melilot Melilotus*

1. The Stalks grow to be three foot high, the Leaves are a Grass green and y Flowers a light Yellow

2. It grows frequently among the Corn and in Hedges, and flowers in June

3. The Leaves and Flowers are accounted mollifying discussing dissolving and easing Pain, for which Uses they are put in Supe and Cataplasms against Inflamations hard Tumours, any kind of Swellings
The Melilot Plaster made of this Herb boiled in Mutton Suet, Rosin and Wax is drawing and good for green Wounds but is chiefly used in Dressing of Blisters
Officinal Preparations are the Emplastrum Melilot simp & Comp

4. Greek Μελιλωτος Latin Melilotus Spanish Corona de Rei. Italian Melilto French Melilot German Zuger Craut Dutch Melilote

5. This Caterpillar is called by some the Hid y Doctor Muffet call it the stage You find it upon most green plants.

10 20

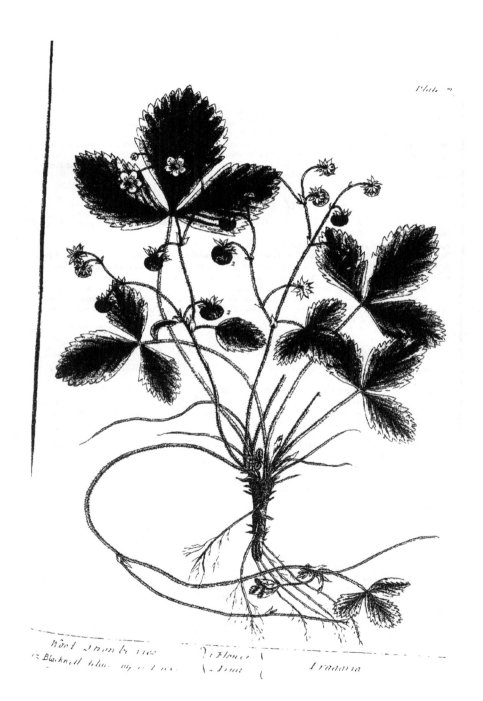

Plate 7

Wood Strawberries
2 Blacknell telius supelta us.   1 Flower   Fradaria
                                    2 Fruit

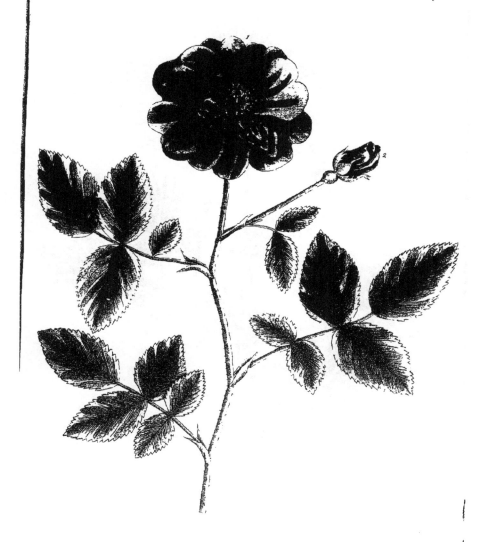

Plate 72

The Red Ro   { 1 Flower }
Eur Pla la h   t q u in   { 2 Bud   }   Rosa rubra

Plate 79

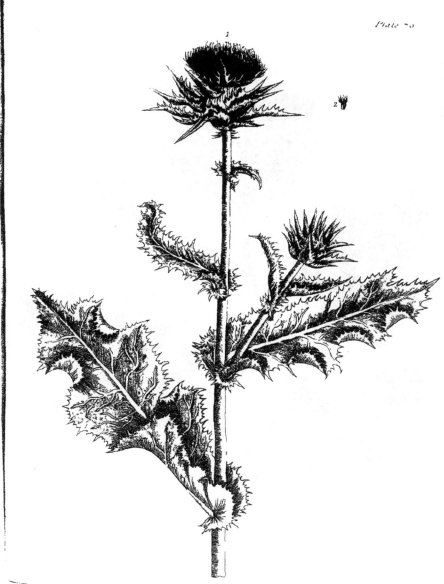

1

2

Ladies Thistle
Eliz: Blackwell delin: sculp: et pinx:

} 1 Flower {
} 2 Seed {

carduus Mariae

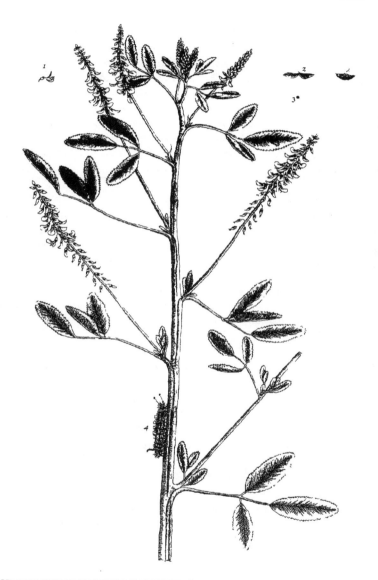

Melilot

Eliz Blackwell delin: sculp: et Pinx

1. *Flower*
2. *Fruit*
3. *Seed*
4. *The Hairy*

Melilotus

Plate 81 Garden Radish Raphanus hortensis

1. The stalks grow to be Three foot high, the Leaves are a dark Green ẏ Flowers are sometimes a light Purple & sometimes white wᵗʰ a red spot on each leaf

2. It is sowen in Gardens, and flowers in May and June

3. Radishes are esteem'd opening attenuating and anuscurbutic They provoke Urine, and are good for the Stone and Gravel.

4. Greek Σαφανίς   Latin, Raphanus   Spanish Ravano   Italian Rafano   French Reffort   German Redich   Dutch   Peperwortel

5. This is called vy Doctor Muffet gryllotalpa or Mole-kricket It lives commonly upon Roots and seldome comes abroad all ẏ Sun is down

---

Plate 82 The Damask Rose   Rosa Damascena

1. This Rose Bush grows not so tall as the white, but taller than the Red, the Leaves are a light Grass green and the Flowers a pale Red

2. It grows in Gardens and flowers for several Months in the Summer

3. The Flowers are of a gentle cathartic Nature purging choleric and serous Humor

They are frequently given to Children & weakly Persons, mixt with stronger Cathartics.

4. Greek Ρόδον   Latin, Rosa Damascena vel pallida   Spanish, Rosas   Italian Rosa French Roses   German Rosen   Dutch, Provincie Roos

---

Plate 83   Pease   Pisum

The stalks grow to be four foot high the Leaves are a very light Green and the Blossomes white

1. They are sowen in Gardens & Fields they flower in May, & ẏ Fruit is ripe in June

2. Pease are accounted good to sweeten ẏ Blood & correct Salt sartine Humor either eaten raw or boiled

3. Greek Πίσος   Latin Pisum   Spanish Arvejas   Italian Piselli & Biso French Les Pois   German Erbsen   Dutch

---

Plate 84   Hedge Nettle   Galeopsis

1. The Stalks grow to be one foot high, ẏ Leaves are a dark green & ẏ Flowers red

2. It grows in Hedges and on Banks and flowers in June

3. This Plant is accounted by some a good vulnerary and serviceable for all sorts of Wounds and putrid Ulcers

It is esteem'd restringent & good to stop inward bleeding & ẏ making of Bloody water

4. Greek Γαλίοψις   Latin Galeopsis   Spanish Ortica muerta   Italian Ortica morta French Ortie   German Daubnessel   Dutch   Doren Netelen

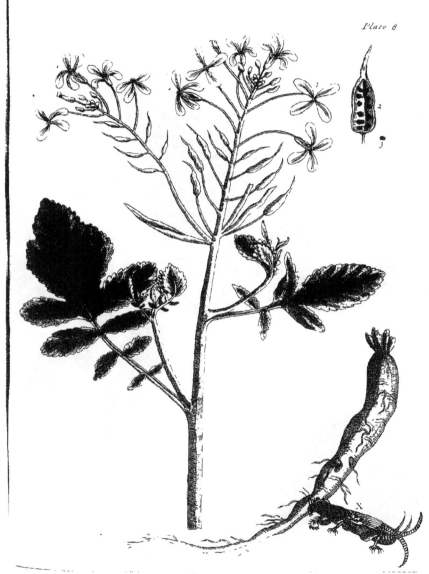

Plate 8

garden Radish

B: Blackwell in   delin   *Raphans hortensis*

Plate 82

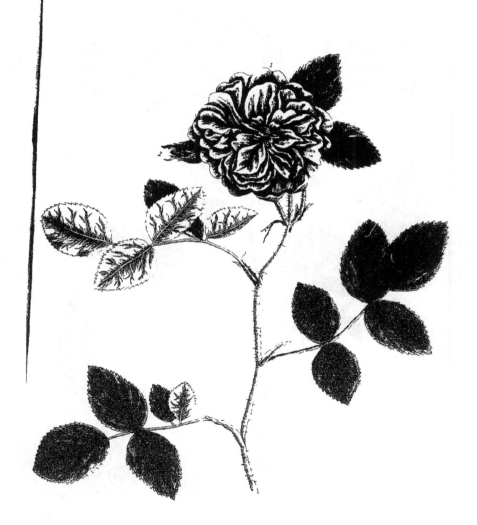

Plate 83

Pea

Blackwell delin calp et Pin   *I. Blossom*   *Pisum*

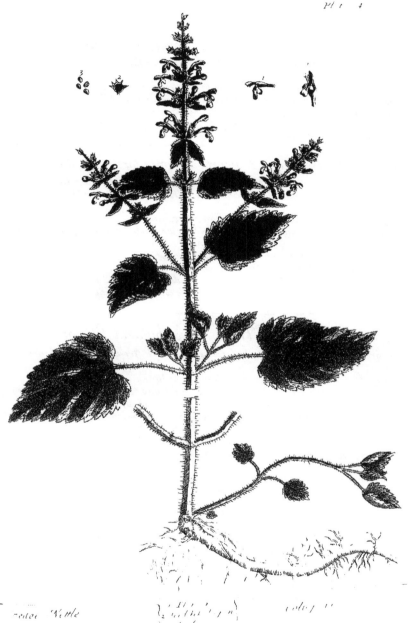

Nettle

Plate 85 Clove July-Flowers. Caryophyllus ruber

The Stalks and Leaves are a light willow Green and the Flowers a fine Red
They are cultivated in Gardens and flower in July
The Flowers are cordial, cephalic and of use in all Diseases of the Head and Nerves
They are used in Fevers and other malignant Distempers, and in Faintings and Palpitations of the Heart
Officinal Preparations are, A Syrup and a Conferve of the Flowers
Greek Καινόφυλλον   Latin Caryophyllus ruber, or tunica vetonica Spanish
Italian Garofoni. French Oeilletz or Girosfloes. German Graſsbltum Dutch.

Plate 86 Water-Betony or Figwort. Scrophularia aquatica

This has larger and taller Stalks than the other Figwort but leſs branch'd and Larger Lea-
ves growing on longer foot Stalks The Leaves and Stalks of this are a Duller Green but the
Flowers a brighter Red
It grows by watery Places and Ditches and flowers in June
It is esteemed good for the Pain and Swelling of the Hæmorrhodes or Piles, and is accounted
by some deterſive and vulnerary and good against the Itch
Greek.   Latin, Scrophularia aquatica, Spanish   Italian Scrofolaria
French Scrolaure German. Wurmeraut Dutch Speenkruyd
This Creature was found by the Side of a Ditch in the middle of June, and since it has lived
Sometimes in water and Sometimes in Earth It eats Herbs and small worms Some think it is a
ſpecies of the Squillae

Plate 87 Great Fig-Wort Scrophularia Major

The Stalks grow to be a Yard high, the Leaves are a graſs Green and the Flowers
a red Purple
It grows in Hedges and Thickets. and flowers in June.
This Plant from the Signature of its Root is accounted good for Scrophulous Tumors
or the Kings Evil in any Part of the Body, as also for the Pain and Swelling of the
Hæmorrhodes, either used inwardly or outwardly it is likewise used for cancerous
stubborn Ulcers
Greek   Latin Scrophularia Major or nodoſe foetida Spanish.
          Italian Scrofolaria French grande Scrolaure German Beyse Ruchtſchatt Dutch
groot Speenkruyd
This Caterpillar is common to both the Figworts, more than any other Plant

Plate 88 . Lettice Lactuca

The Stalks grow to be two or three foot high, the Leaves us a light green and the Flowers yellow
It is sown in Gardens and flowers according to the Months it is sown in
Lettice is generally the Principal Ingredient in Sallets being grateful to the Stomach allay
ing Heat, quenching Thirst, and temper the Sharpneſs of Humors in the Body it provok
Urine, and encreaſes Milk in Nurſes
The Seed is one of the four smaller cold Seeds
Greek Θειδ'αζ Latin Lactuca Spanish Lechuga Italian Lattuca French Laucue
German Lattich Dutch Salade

No 22

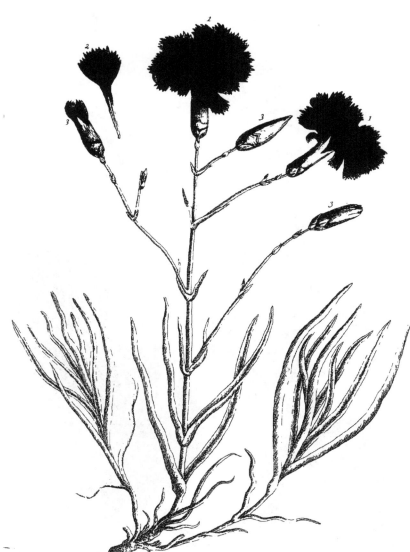

Plate 85

Clove July Flower
Blacknell White coloured Pink
1 Flower
2 Flower separate
3 Bud
caryophyllus rutus

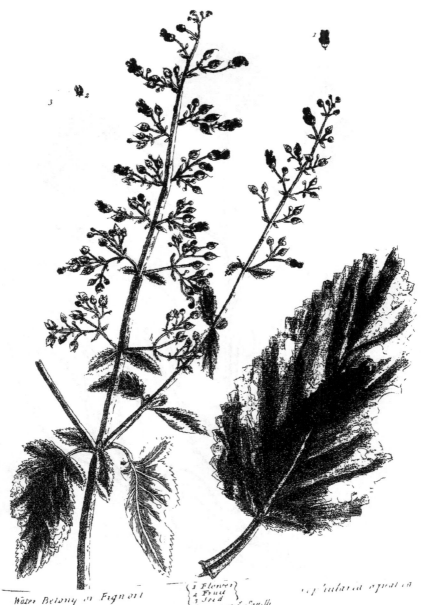

3   2   1

Water Betony or Figwort   { 1 Flower }   Scrophularia aquatica
                             { 2 Fruit }
                             { 3 Seed   }

Eliz. Blackwell delin.   sculp. et Pinx.

Plate 7.

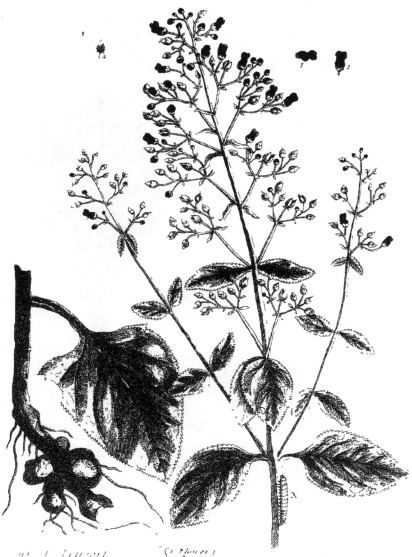

2 Fruit
3 Seed

Scrophularia major

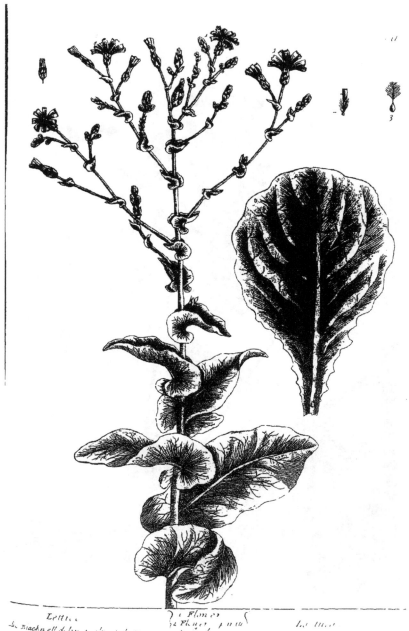

Plate 89 Bears Breech, or Brank Ursin. Acanthus Branca Ursina.

The Stalks grow to be two foot high. the Leaves are a shining dark Green colour, the Flowers are white

It is said that the Ancients took the Pattern of their foliage Work from the Leaves of this Plant

It is cultivated here in Gardens, its native Place being Italy Spain and the Southern Part of France :
Flowers in July

This Plant is used in Glisters and Baths for Obstructions and for the Stone and Gravel

The Herb Women sell the Leaves of the Helleboraster or Bears foot or Sphondylium or Cow parsnep
instead of this Plant to those that are ignorant

Greek Ακανθος Latin. Acanthus Branca Ursina or Acanthus sativus Spanish Yerva giguante and
branqua Ursina. Italian Acantho or Branca Orsina French, Branxe Orsine German Beren Aan Dutch
This Moth was produced from the Caterpillar Plate 76

Plate 90 Marshmallows Althaea Bismalva, Ibiscus

The Stalks grow to be a Yard high the Leaves are of a yellowish green Colour the Flowers are a
pale Red

It grows in Salt Marshes and flowers in July

This Plant is mollifying digesting and Soupling of great use in the Strangury Gravel Stone Heat
of Urine corroding Humors in the Stomach and Guts Coughs Hoarsness Swellings & Inflamations

Officinal Preparations are, the Syrupus de Althea, Pulv: Dialtheæ & Unguentum Dialtheæ

Greek Αλθεια & Εβιοκος Latin Althaea. Bismalva Ibiscus Spanish Hierva Caunamera or Mar
nage Italian. Malvavischio French Guymauve German Ibisch Dutch Heemswortel

---

Plate 91 Great Celandine or Yellow-horn Poppy Chelidonium majus

The Stalks grow to be a foot high. the Leaves are a bluish Green and the Flowers yellow

It grows among waste Grounds and Rubbish, and upon old Walls it flowers in May and June

It is accounted apperative and cleansing, opening Obstructions of the Spleen & Liver, &
of great Use in Curing y Jaundice and Scurvy — Some reckon it cordial & good against
pestilential Distempers . — Outwardly for sore Eyes to dry up the Rheum, and to
take an ay Specks, Films, Tetters, Ringworms & Scurfy Breakings-out

Greek Χελιδονιον μεγα Latin Chelidonium majus, or Papaver Corniculatum luteum
Spanish, Celiduena, or Yerva dellas Golundrinas Italian Celidonia maggiore French,
Cheledoine as Eschlere German, Schelscraut Dutch, Sankende Byrone

---

Plate 92 Goats Rue Galega, or Ruta caprana

The Stalks grow to be a Yard high, the Leaves are a grass Green, & y Flowers a pale Blue
L grows in several Places of Italy wild, but is planted here in Gardens and flowers
in June and July

Goats Rue is esteem'd cordial, sudorific, alexipharmic good against pestilential Distem
pers - It is also of use in most Fevers, the Small Pox and Measels — It kills H r
and is good to cure the Bites of Venemous Creatures

Greek   Latin Galega or Ruta capraria Spanish
Italian.   French.   German
Dutch

No 23

Plate 30

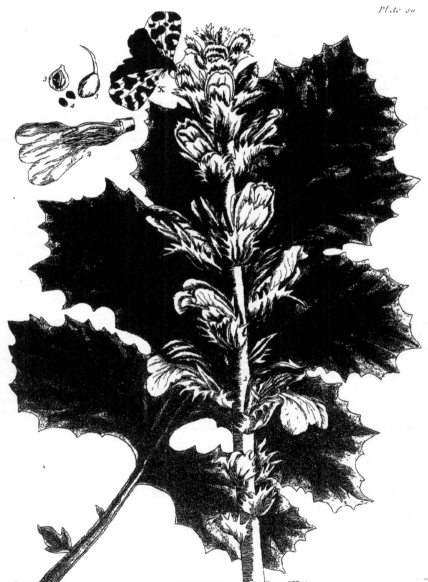

Bears Breech or brank Ursine

Acanthus branca Ursina

Brank Ursine of the shops

Acre or Leopard

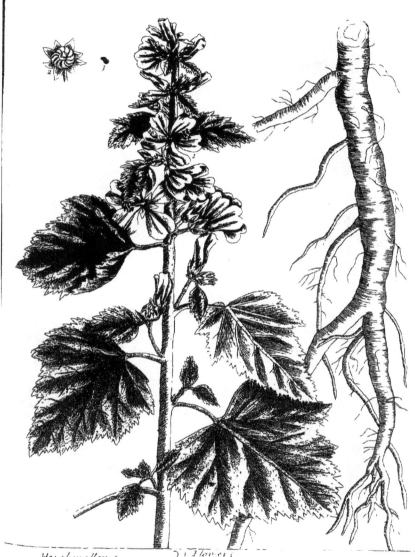

Marshmallow

1 Flower
2 Fruit
3 Seed

Althaea Bismalva Ibiscus

Plate 91

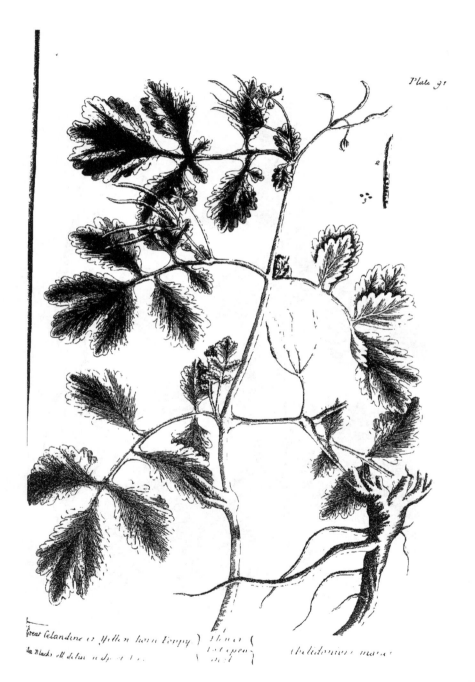

Great Celandine or Yellow horn Poppy.   Chelidonium majus
the Black Oil delin & Sculp

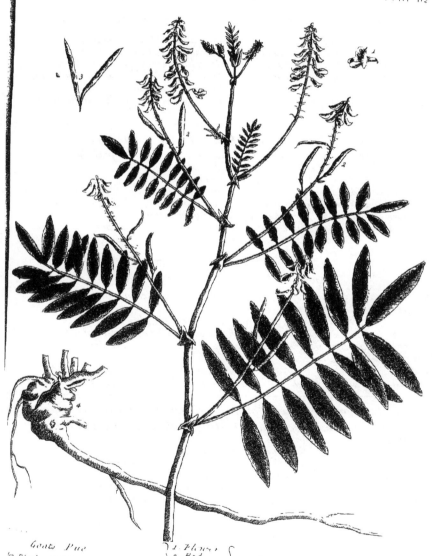

Plate 62

Goats Rue

Blackwell delin Sculp et Pinx

1 Flower
2 Pod
3 Pod open
4 Root

Galeca or Ruta capraria

Plate 93 Great Centory Centaurium majus, or magnum
1 The Stalks grow to be five or six foot high the Leaves are a light Green and the Flowers purplish
2 It grows wild in Italy but is planted here in Gardens and flowers in July
3 The Root is accounted drying, binding good for all kinds of Fluxes stopping Bleeding at the Nose, Mouth. or any other Part. - It is also esteemed good to heal Wounds taking its Name as Pliny says from the Centaur Chiron who cured himself of a Wound he received by one of the Arrows of Hercules, by the Use of this Plant
4 Greek Κενταύριον μέγα Latin Centaurium magnum Spanish Ruipontie Italian Centaurea maggiore French Rhepontico German Reupontict Dutch.

Plate 94 Tutsan or Park Leaves Androsaemum
1 The Stalks grow to be two or three foot high the Leaves are a grass Green the Flowers Yellow, and the Berries when ripe purple
2 It grows in Hedges and Thickets and flowers in July
3 The Leaves and Flowers are accounted much of the Nature of St John's Wort being a good Wound Herb used both inwardly and outwardly - In French it is called Toutsain, All heal, and from thence by us corruptly Tutsan
4 Greek Ἀνδρόσαιμον Latin Androsaemum - vulgare - Clymenon Spanish Italian Androsemo French, Toutsain German Dutch,

---

Plate 95 Thorow-Wax Perfoliata
1 It grows to be a foot high, the Leaves are a blue Green, and the Flowers a greenish Yellow
2 It grows among the Corn, and flowers in June & July
3 Thorough Wax is reckond among the Vulnerary Plants and is much used for green Wounds Bruises Ruptures Contusions old Ulcers and Sores, either given in Powder or the Decoction
4 Greek. Latin Perfoliata - vulgaris Spanish Italian Perfogliata French German Durchwaßhß Dutch

---

Plate 96 Swallow-Wort Tame Poison Asclepias-Vincetoxicum ẽ Hirundinaria
1 The Stalks are about a foot and a half high the Leaves are a dark grass Green, and the Flowers white
2 It grows here in Gardens and flowers in June and July
3 The Root is esteemed a great Counterpoison especially against the bad Effects of Apocynum. and other poisonous Herbs.
It is also used to cure the Stings and Bites of Venemous Creatures.
It is helpful against Malignant pestilential Fevers which it carries off by Sweat
It is used also for the Dropsie and Jaundice.
Greek Ἀσκληπιάς Latin Asclepias Spanish   Italian Vincetoßico.
French   German Schwallenwurt Dutch,

Plate 93

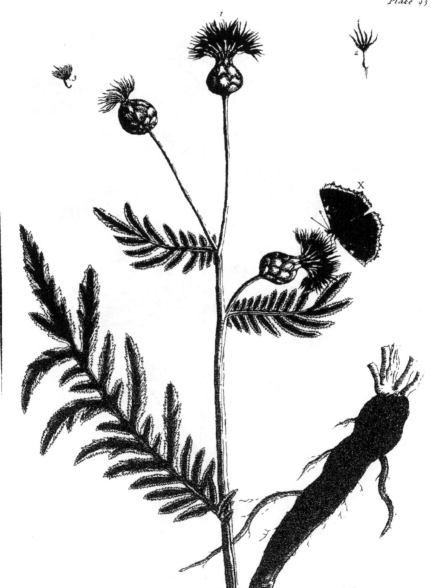

great centory

Eliz Blackwell delin. sulp et Pinx

1 Flower
2 Flower separate
3 Seed
X the Urchin Moth

centaurium majus or magnum

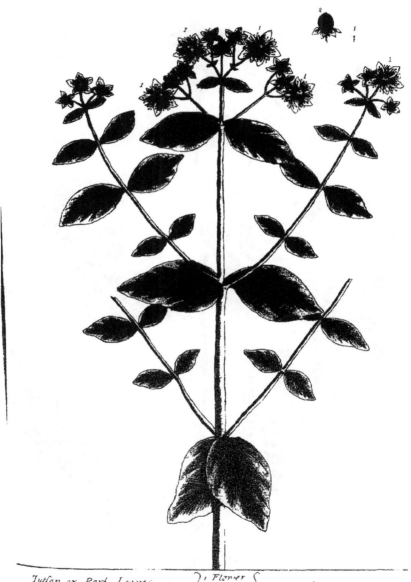

Tusan or Park Leaues.

Eliz Blackwell delin sculp et Pinx

1 Flower
2 Fruit
3 Seed

Androsaemum.

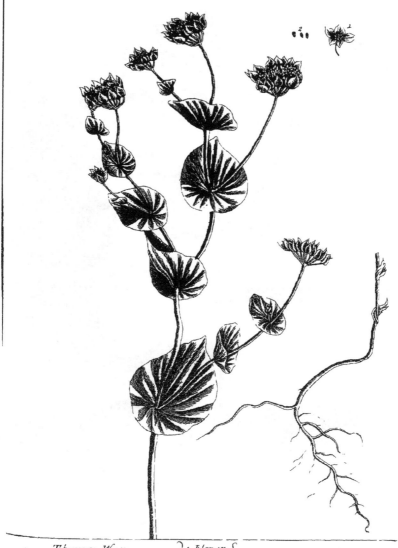

Plate 95

Thoron Wax   1 Flower   Perfoliata

Fliz. Blackwell delin. sculp. et Pinx.   2 Seed

Plate 102

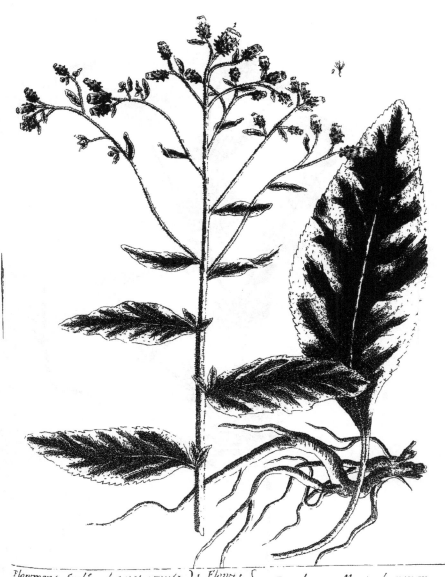

Flowmans Spikenard great tougst {1 Flower} Baccharis Monspeliensium
Var Blackwell delin culs et Pinx {2 Seed}

Plate 1

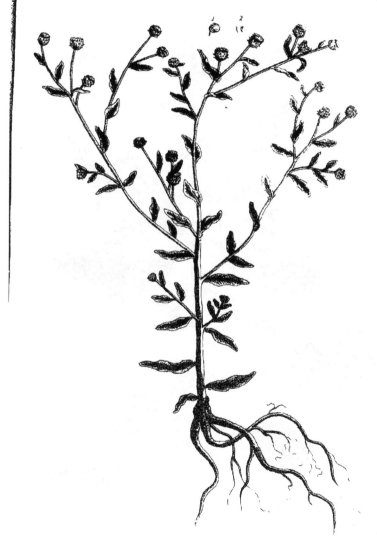

Flea bane

Eliz Blackwell delin. sculp. et Pinx —

{ 1 Flower {
{ 2 Seed { ..onyza and Pulicaria

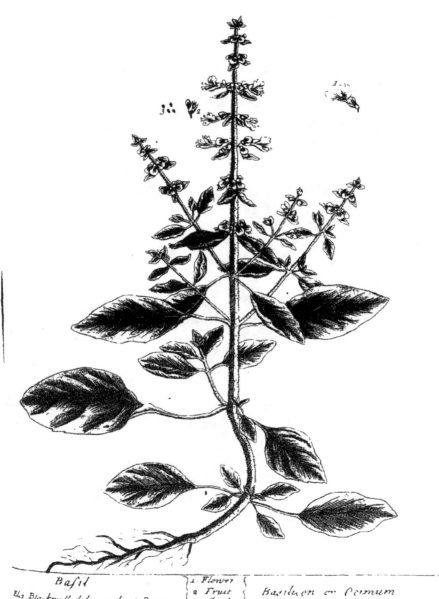

Basil

1. Flower
2. Fruit
3. Seed

Basilicon or Ocimum

Plate 105 The Almond Tree Amygdalus

1. This Tree resembles that of the Peach in the Leaves and Blossomes, only the Blossomes in this are paler
2. The Almond Tree is a Native of Spain and Barbary, it flowers early in ye Spring and the Fruit is ripe in August
3. Sweet Almonds are accounted nourishing, but if eaten too much hard of Digesting The Oil of the Sweet is good in Affections of the Lungs, Stone Gravel collic. It is good for Women to take freely of it before they Expect their Delivery, and of great Service to purge Children mixed with any opening Syrup The Bitter are used as a Cosmetic, being cleansing and beautifying The Oil dropt into the Ears is good for Deafness, & is frequently put among Anodine Liniments The Officinal Preparations are the Expressed Oils
4. greek Αμυγδαλος Latin Amygdalus, amara & dulcis sativa Spanish Almendras Italian Mandrole French Amandes German Mandelbaum Dutch Amandelroom

---

Plate 106 Marygolds. Calendula.

1. The Leaves are a light Green and the Flowers Yellow
2. It grows in Gardens, and flowers great part of the Summer
3. The Leaves and Flowers are accounted Cordial Alexipharmice good in all kinds of Feavers, they promote sweat and are frequently used to drive out the small Pox and Measles Some commend them for the Jaundice, sore Inflamed Eyes, and Warts
4. Greek   Latin. Calendula. simplice flore. maxima talcha vulgaris Spanish   Italian Fior Rancio French Poulsy German Ringel Idum Dutch Bouldbloem.

Plate 107 Night-Shade Solanum hortense

1. It grows to se 2 foot high, the Leaves are a grass Green, and the Flowers White with a Yellow Umba in the Middle
2. It grows by High Ways, and among Rubbish, and Flowers in August
3. The Flower and Leaves are used, and esteem'd cooling good for all kinds of Inflammations and hot Swellings, the Shingles and other cuticular Eruptions as also for Burns and Scalds This is the Solanum that should be put in the Unguentum Populeon, but the Herb folks sell the Solanum lignosum in it stead, which is of a contrary Nature, therefore it is better to use the Solanum lethale which is to be had at the same time, and agrees better with ye other Ingredients
4. Greek Στρύχνος κηπαιος   Latin Solanum hortense – vulgare. Spanish. Yerva mora Italian Salato o or Herbamorella French. Morelle German Nachtschatt Dutch Nachtschade

---

Plate 108 Wild Cucumber Cucumis agrestis afininus

1. The Stalk of this Plant creep on the Ground, the Leaves are a light Green and the Flowers Yellow
2. It is sown in Gardens here, and flower in July
3. This is a Strong Cathartic, carrying off serous watery Humors both upwards and downwards with great Violence, whence it is of great Use in the Dropsy when ye Bowles are not decayed, it forcibly brings down the Catamena and even destroys the Foetus in the Womb so it is therefore only fit to be administred by a very skilful Hand.
4. Greek. Σικυs αγριος   Latin, Cucumis sylvestris – asininus Spanish Cogombrillos amargos Italian. Cocomero salvatico French. Cogombre asinia German. Bilder Cucumer Dutch Esels Comcommer

No 27

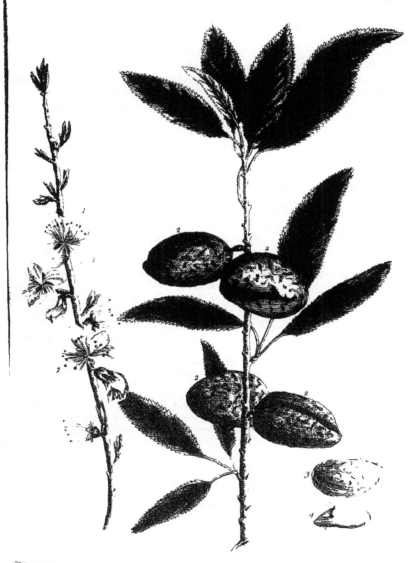

Plate 1

The Almond Tree

Eliz. Blackwell delin. sculp et Pinx.

1 Blossome
2 Fruit
3 Stone
4 Kernel

Amygdalus

Plate 110

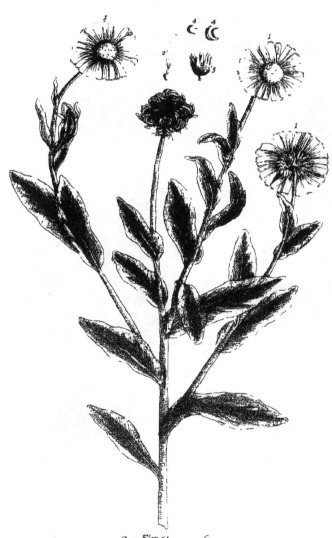

Marygold
Eliz Blackwell delin. sculp. et Pinx

1. Flower
2. Flower apart
3. calix
4. Root

Calendula

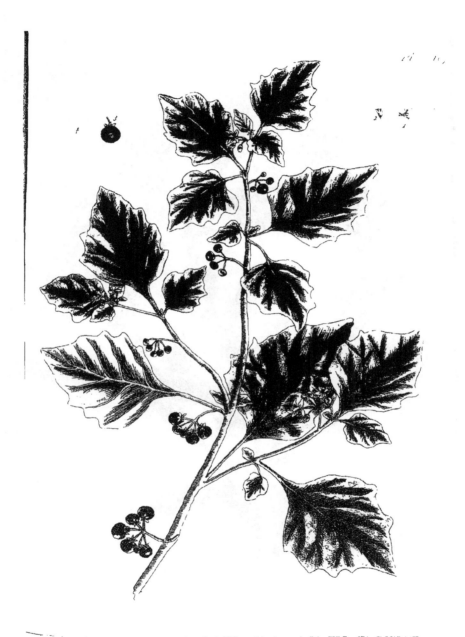

Night Shade   Solanum Dulcamara

Plate 105

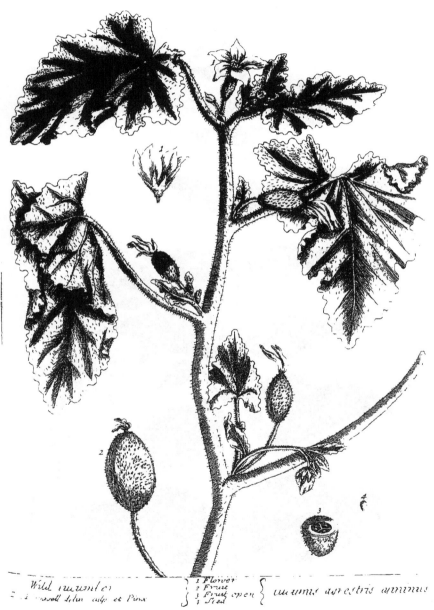

Wild cucumber

1 Flower
2 Fruit
3 Fruit open
4 Seed

cucumis agrestis minimus

Plate 96

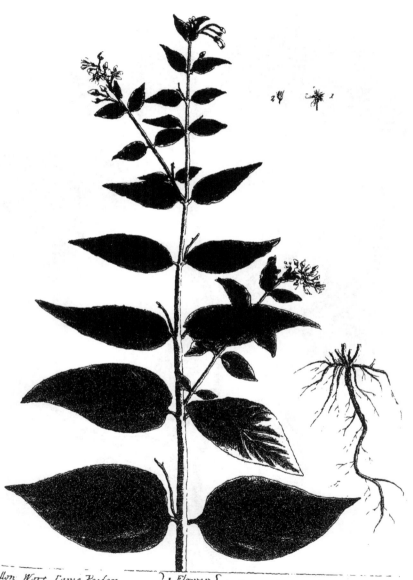

Swallon Wort Tame Poison

Eliz Blackwell delin s ulp et Pinx

1 Flower
2 Calix

Asclepias Vincetoxicum & Hirundinaria

Plate 97 Pomgranates granata, Punica mala

, This is a low Tree having on its Branches a few Thorns. The Leaves are a fine Grass Green and the Flowers a fine Scarlet

₂ Pomgranates grow in Spain & Italy and many other Countries, and flower in June and July

₃ The Balustia off are the large double Flowers of ẙ wild Pomgranate, which differs not in its manner of Growth from the other, These, as well as the single Flowers, and the Bark are very drying & restringent good for all sorts of Fluxes, Hemorrhages, Bleedings They strengthen the Gums fasten loose Teeth help the falling down of the Uvula and cancerous Ulcers in the Mouth and Throat

₄ Greek ρόια Latin Granata Spanish Granadas Italian Melagrano or Pomo granato French Pomes de Grenades or Mygrains German, Granatopffelbaum Dutch Granaat Boom

Plate 98 Costmary or Alecoast Balsamita mas or Costus hortorum

₁ The Stalks grow to be more than a foot high the Leaves are a yellow Green and the Flowers yellow

₂ It is planted in Gardens and Flowers in July

₃ The Leaves are accounted good to strengthen the Stomach & ease ẙ Head ᾰch arising from the Disorders thereof — It expells Wind and prevents sour Belchings outwardly it is used in Fomentations to comfort and strengthen the Limbs

₄ Greek   Latin Costus hortorum Spanish   Italian Menta Greca French, Coch German, Buser Frauen Munk Dutch Balsame

Plate 99 Arrach Atriplex.

₁ The Stalks grow to be 3 foot high the Leaves are a pale Green and sometimes purplish, and the Flowers a greenish yellow

₂ It grows in Gardens and flowers in June and July

₃ The Leaves are frequently boiled & eaten like coleworts with Salt Meats & in Sallads and are esteem'd cooling and moistning rendring the Body soluble, and good for hot bilious Constitutions — They are used with other emollient Herbs in cooling Clisters

₄ Greek ᾰτραφαξις Latin Atriplex - alba hortensis - pallida viriens Spanish Armoles Italian Atriplice French Arroches German Molten Dutch Melde

Plate 100 Wild stinking Arrach Atriplex olida.

The Stalks of this Plant spread on the Ground and the Leaves are covered with a mealy Green, the Flowers are small and Green The whole Plant has a strong foetid fishy Smell

₂ It grows on Dunghills & Waste Places flowring for some Months in the Summer

₃ This Herb is peculiarly appropriated to ẙ female Sex, being operative deobstruent usefull in uterine Disorders good to promote the Menses expell ẙ Afterbirth help childbed Purgations, appease ẙ Strangulations of ẙ Womb, take ẙ hasten ẙ Fits It is usually given in a Decoction There is a Syrup kept in ẙ Shops made with ẙ Juce of this Plant & Sugar

₄ Greek Ατάφαξις αγρια Latin Atriplex olida - silvestris Spanish Armoles Italian Reppice Salvatico French Arroches sauvages German Bild Molten Dutch Bild Melde

No 25

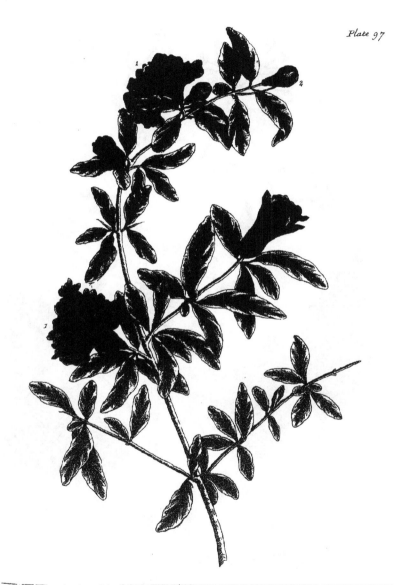

Plate 97

Pomgranate

L. Blackwell delin.

1 Flower
2 Bud

Granata Punica mala

Plate 98

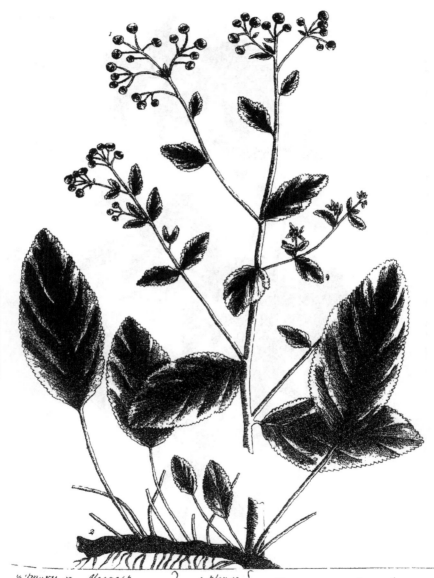

Costmary or Alecoast

1 Flower
2 Part of ye Fruit

Ballsmita ma[?] Costus hortorum

E. Blackwell delin: sculp: et Pinx:

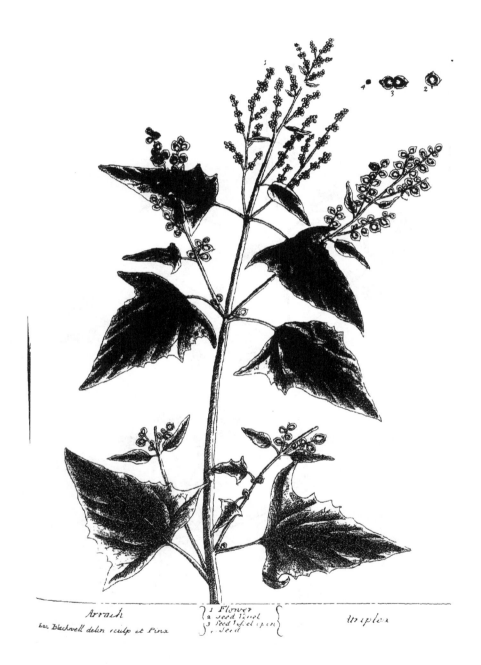

Arrach

Eliz: Blackwell delin sculp et Pinx

1 Flower
2 Seed Vessel
3 Seed Vessel open
4 Seed

Atriplex

Plate 100

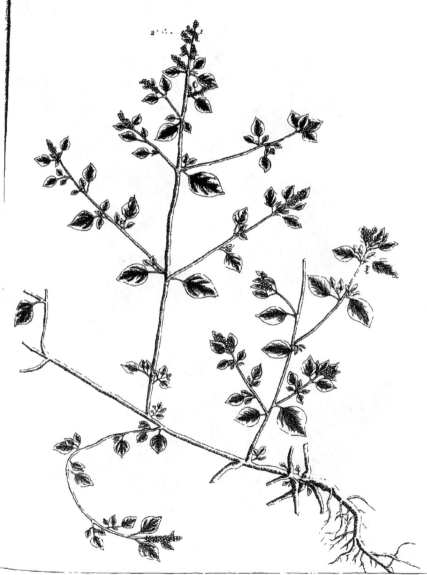

Wild stinking Arrach

Eliz Blackwell delin sculp et Pinx

} 1 Flower {
} 2 Seed {

Atriplex olida

Plate 101 The Peach Tree Perfica Malus

1 This Tree grows to no great Bigness here the Leaves are a deep green. and the Flowers a fine Pink Colour

2 It is planted in Gardens & flowers in March, the Fruit is ripe in August

3 The Flowers are opening and purging, and are chiefly given to Children to carry off their serous Humors, and to kill Worms The Fruit is cooling and moistning gratefull to the Palate, but apt to putrefy and cause Surfeits

4 Greek τεροικα μηλα, and Ποδακηνα Latin Perfica Malus Spanish, Pexegos Italian Pefiche & Perfiche French. Pefches German Pferfich Dutch.

Plate 102 Plowmans Spikenard great Conyfa Baccharis Monfpeliensium

1 The Stalks grow to be Three foot high, the Leaves are a dull Green and the Flowers Yellow

2 It grows on hilly chalky Places and flowers in July

3 This Plant is esteemed by some a good Vulnerary, for Bruises Contufions Ruptures and Inward Wounds Pains in ÿ Side & Difficulty of Breathing

4 Greek Ko . . Latin Baccharis Monfpeliensium, and Conyfa major vulgaris Spanish Altadegua Italian Coniza or Pulicaria French. Herbe aux Puces . . . Geel Munk Dutch,

Plate 103 Flea-bane Conyfa & Pulicaria.

1 The . . . . about a Span high, the Leaves are a grafs Green and the Flowers yellow

2 It grows in moist Places, and where Water has stood all the Winter, and flowers in August and September

3 This is the Pulicaria of Lobel so call'd because by its Smell it deftroys Fleas and . . . Parkinfon and Gerard commend the Conyfa Media as better than this Some . . . . . intment made of this Plant as good for the Itch

4 Greek . . . . . Latin Conyfa and Pulicaria Spanish, Altadequa menore Italian . . . . French Herb aux Puces German, Geel Munk Dutch

Plate 104 Basil Basilicon or Ocimum.

1 It grows about a foot high the Leaves are a light Green and the Flowers white

2 It is sown in gardens and flowers in July and August

3 The Ancients condemn the inward ufe of this Plant as hurtfull to the Sight Schroder commends it as good to cleanse ÿ Lungs of Flegm and provoke the Menfes The Leaves are ufed in the Aq Hysterica and Ung Martiatum The Seed is ufed in the Aq Vitæ comp Syrup Artemisiæ Puh Diarrhodon See Casper Commelin p 56

4 Greek Ωκιμον Latin Basilicon & Ocimum Spanish Albahaca Italian Basilico French Basilic German Basilien Dutch Basilicon

Nᵒ 26

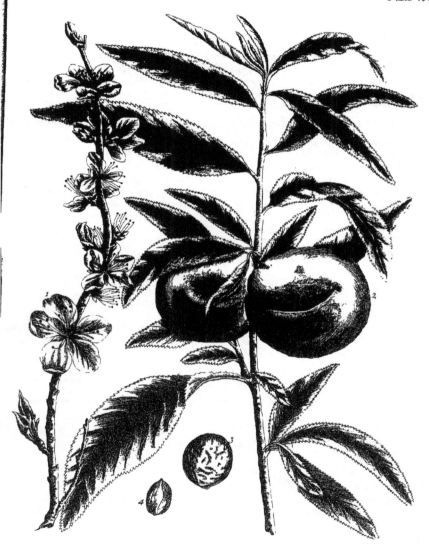

Plate 101

The Peach Tree

Ehe Blackwell delin sculp et Pinx

{ 1 Flower
2 Fruit
3 the Stone
4 the Kernel {

Persica Malus

Plate 109 *Starwort, or Aster Attic. Aster Atticus or Inguinalis*

1 The stalks grow to be a foot and an half high, the Leaves are a Grass Green, & the Flowers purple with a Yellow Thrum in the Middle

2 It is planted here in Gardens, its native place being Greece, Italy, Spain, & the Southern Parts of France. It flowers in August

3 The Ancients commended the Leaves, beaten & applyed as a Cataplasm, against Buboes and Swellings in the Groin

Dioscorides recommends it for the too great Heat of y Stomach, & Inflammations of the Eyes

4 Greek, Ασης ἀτλικός Latin, Aster Atticus, Inguinalis or Bubonium Spanish Astaraticon Italian, Asteratico French, Petite Espargoutte German, Stern Graut Dutch

---

Plate 110 *The Eupatorium of Avicenna. Eupatorium Avicennae*

1 The Stalks grow to be two or three foot high, the Leaves are a light Grass Green, & the Flowers purplish.

2 It grows by Rivers and Ditches and flowers in August.

3 Schroder commends this as a very good Vulnerary Plant, used inwardly, but especially outwardly; & useful to correct an Ill Habit of Body, & cure Coughs & Catarrhs

4 Greek. Latin, Eupatorium Avicenna or vulgare Spanish, Agrimonia Italian, Eupatorio French, German, Curugundt Graut Dutch,

---

Plate 111 *White Henbane. Hyoscyamus albus.*

1 The Stalks grow to be two Foot high, the Leaves are a dark Green, and the Flowers a pale Yellow

2 It is a Native of the warm Countries, being planted with us in Gardens, flowring in July and August

3. This Henbane is accounted milder than the Black and therefore safer to be given inwardly, being emollient cooling and Anodyne, good for Inflamations, and Defluctions of hot Rheum, and is often put into cooling repelling Ointments

4 Greek, Υοσκίαμος λευκός Latin, Hyoscyamus albus Spanish, Velenho blanco Italian, Iusquiamo branco French, Iusquiame blanc German, Bilsam Dutch, Bilsenkryd.

Plate 112 *Alkanet. Anchusa.*

1 The Stalks grow about two foot high, the Leaves are a dark Green, and the Flowers a blue Purple

2 It grows in Gardens here, and flowers in June and July.

3 Dioscorides & other Ancients commend the Root as good against the Bites of Venemous Creatures being drank in Wine, - & outwardly against Burns & St Anthony's Fire, - Parkinson commends the Infusion of the Bark in Petroleum as good for fresh Cuts and green Wounds

4 Greek, Άγχ εσα ἑτέρα Latin, Anchusa. Spanish Sagem. Italian, Anchusa. French, Orchanette German, Rot Ochfenjungen Dutch Alkanne.

No 28.

Plate 109

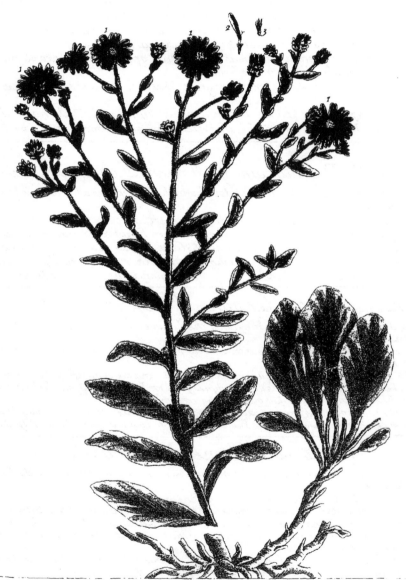

Starwort or Aster attic

The Blackwell delin. sculp et Pinx

1 Flower
2 Flower separate
3 Seed

Aster atticus or Inguinalis

Plate 110

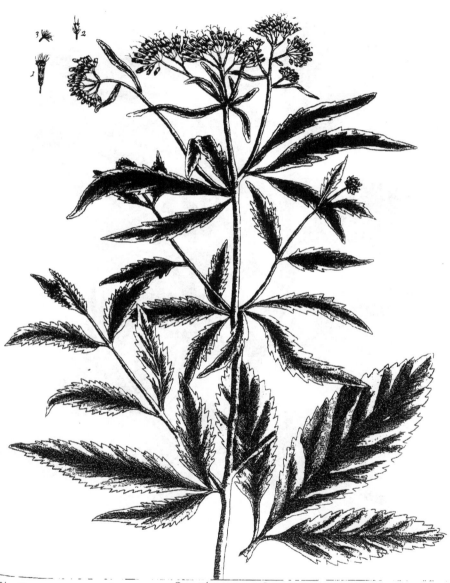

The Eupatorium of Avicenna

Eliz. Blackwell delin. sculp. et Pinx

1 Flower
2 Flower separate
3 Seed

Eupatorium Avicenae

Plate 111

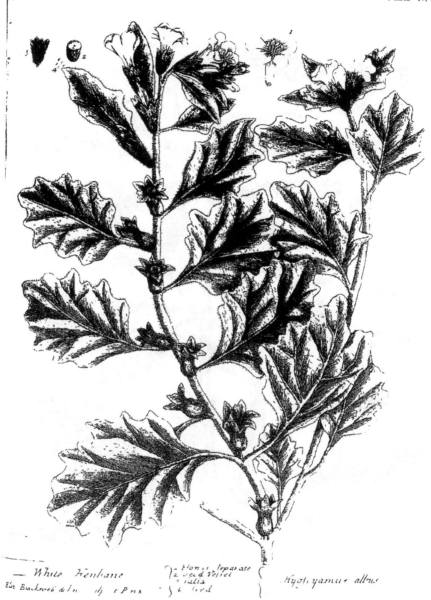

— White Henbane

E.a: Blackwell a l.n.   d, t P.n.x

1. Flon s separate
2. Seed Vessel
3. alia
4. seed

Hyos,yamus albus

Plate 112

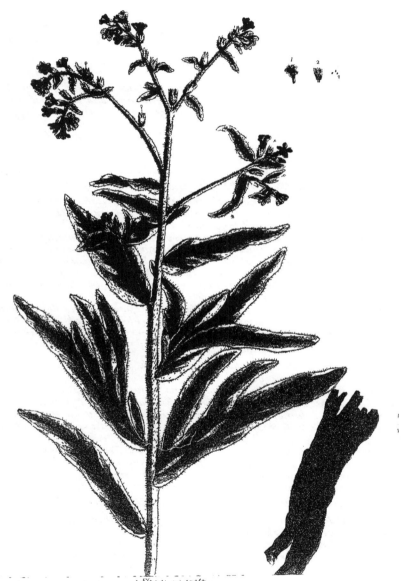

Alkanet
Anchusa officinalis sp. Linn.
1 Flores magnato
2 tur

Plate 113 Sopewort or Brusewort *Saponaria* - Vulgaris

1. It grows to be a foot and an half high, the Leaves are a grass Green, and the Flowers a pale Purple
2. It grows in Watery Places near Rivers and flowers for several Months in the Summer
3. It is called Saponaria, or Sopewort, because its Juice will get greasy Spots out of Cloaths It is esteemed opening and attenuating and somewhat sudorific It is recommended by some against the Lues Venerea - Outwardly applied it helps hard Tumours and Whitlows
4. Greek, Λυχνις Latin, Saponaria vulgaris, or Lychnis Saponaria dicta Spanish, Italian, Lichnide coronaria French, German, Margenroslin Dutch, Seepkruyd

Plate 114 The Mirtle Tree *Myrtus - Bœtica sylvestris*

1. This is a little Tree shooting forth many slender tough Branches, the Leaves of which are a grass Green, and the Flowers White
2. It grows wild in Spain and Italy, flowring in August
3. The Leaves as well as the Berries are accounted drying & binding, good for a Diarrhœa or Dysentery spitting of Blood, catarrhous Defluxions upon the Breast the Fluor albus, the falling down of the Womb or Fundament, both taken inwardly - Outwardly they are used in Powders & Injections Preparations from y Berries are Syrupus Myrtinus Pul Diamargariton frigid Ol Myrtinum Ung adstringens Kernel Empl ad Rupturas
4. Greek, μυρσινη Latin Myrtus Spanish Murta, or Rayam Italian Myrto mortana & Mortella French Meurte German, Belsckheiderbeer baum Dutch Myrte Boom

Plate 115 Toad-Flax *Linaria* - lutea vulgaris

1. The Stalks grow a little more than a foot high, the Leaves are a willow green, and the Flowers Yellow
2. It grows common on Banks and Hedges and flowers in Iuly
3. The whole Plant is used, being accounted diuretic opening Obstructions of the Liver & Spleen, helping the Dropsy and Iaundice which it carries off by Urine The Ointment made with Hoggs Lard and a good Quantity of this Herb, is esteemed a good Remedy of the Piles by anointing the Part, - at the time of Using it mix some of y Yolk of an Egg with it - The Officinal Preparation is y Ung Linariæ
4. Greek Ουρις Latin Linaria - lutea vulgaris and Osyris Spanish, Linaria, Italian Linaria French Linaire German Harnkraut Dutch.

Plate 116 Tarragon *Dracunculus hortensis*

1. It grows to be two foot high the Leaves are a shineing dark Green and the Flowers a Yellowish colour
2. It is planted in Gardens, and flowers in Iuly and August
3. The Leaves which are chiefly used are accounted heating and drying good for those who have cold Stomachs, for which they are often put into Sallads, - Some say they expell Wind, provoke Urine & the Menses
4. Greek, Latin Dracunculus hortensis Spanish Dragono Italian Dragone French, Targon German Dragunell Dutch Dragon

Plate 111

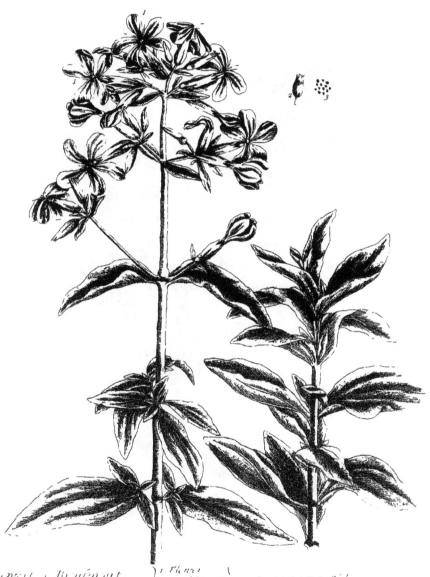

Soapwort. Bruisewort.   1 Fleur.   Saponaria officinalis.
Bluejacket de l'une et l'autre.   2 med vessell.
                                     3 seed.

Plate 114

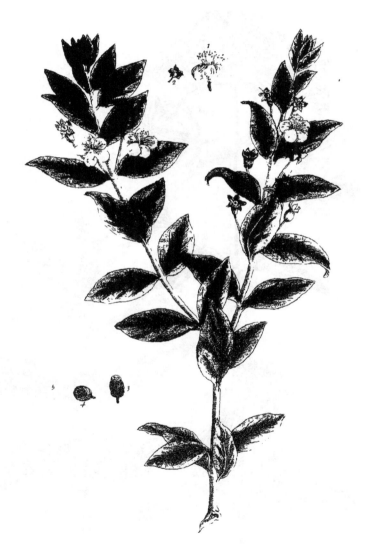

The Myrtle Tree

Plate 115

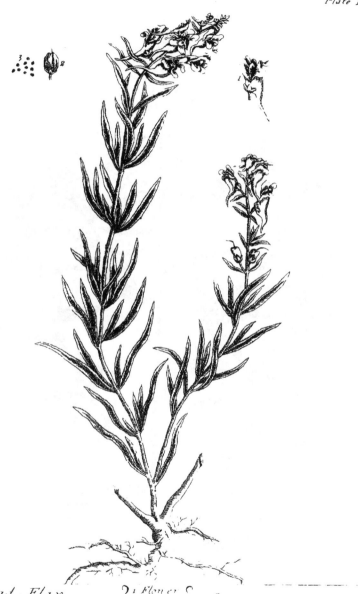

Toad-Flax

Ez Blackwell delin sculp et Pinx

1 *Flower*
2 *Fruit*
3 *Seed*

Linaria lutea vulgaris.

Plate 116

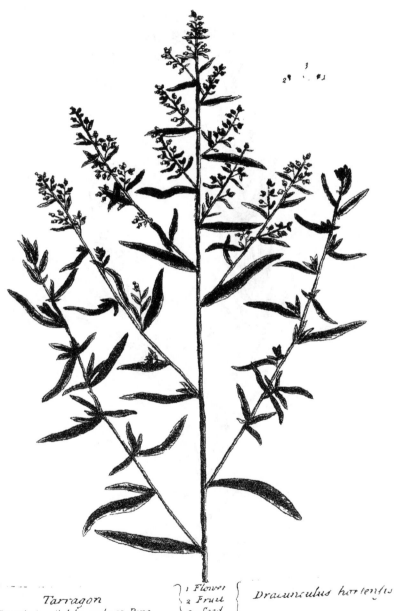

Tarragon
Fuz Blackwell delin sculp et Pinx

{ 1 Flower
2 Fruit
3 Seed }

Dracunculus hortensis

Plate 117 The great Burdock   Bardana major Lappa major

1 The stalks grow to be two Foot high, the Leaves are white & hoary underneth, and a deep grass Green above, and the Flowers are Purple

2 It grows by Way sides and flowers in Iune and Iuly.

3 The Roots are sudorific and alexapharmic good in malignant Fevers, & are therefore used in the Aq Theriacalis - They are accounted good against the Gout and Pains in ÿ Limbs - The Leaves boild in Milk, and applied as a Cataplasm are by some used for the same Distemper, as also for Burns and Inflammations, and are one of the Ingredients of the Unguent Populneum - The common People apply them often to ÿ Feet & Wrists in Fevers - The Seed powderd and given in white Wine is good to provoke Urine, and help Fits of the Stone

4 Greek. Ἄρκτιον Latin Bardana, Personata or Lappa major Spanish Bardana Italian, Lappola maggiore French. Glisteron or Bardana German Gross Pletten. Dutch. Klitsen

Plate 118 Dead or spotted Arsmart Persicaria maculata or maculosa

1 It grows to be two Foot high, the Leaves are a deep Green with a spot in ÿ middle in shape like a half Moon and the Flowers are a pale Red

2 It grows in moist Places by Ponds and Ditches and flowers in Iuly

3 The Leaves are esteemd by some of a cooling Nature good against hot Tumors Inflammations, Imposthumes and green Wounds

4 Greek. Ὑδροπέπερι Latin Persicaria maculosa Spanish Hierva pexequiera Italian Persicaria maggiore French Curage German Schmecken Dutch Persich - kruyd

Plate 119 Sharp Arsmart or Water Pepper Hydropiper

1 This Plant grows to the same height as the former, the Leaves are lighter and want the spot in the dead Arsmart and the Flowers are a paler Red

2 It grows in the same Places as the other, and flowers at the same time

3 The great Mr Boyle in his Book of the Usefulness of Experimental Phylosophy recommends the distilld Water of this Plant as a good Remedy against the Stone It is commended also as very cleansing and good for old stubborn Ulcers

4 Greek Ὑδροπέπερι Latin Hydropiper and Persicaria   maculata Spanish Hierva manchas Italian Pepe aquatico and Persicaria French Curage German Baserpfeffer Dutch Persuh kruyd

Plate 120 Buckshorn or Swines Cresses Coronopus Ruellii

1 The lower Leaves of this Plant lie on the Ground, and are in shape and colour like the Garden Cresses, the Flowers are White

2 It grows by Way Sides and flowers great Part of the Summer

3 In the West Country this is much used as a Sallad both raw and boiled, for its great Usefulness in the Stone and Gravel, and several gardners about London cultivate it in their Gardens for this End being a great diuretic

4 Greek.   Latin Coronopus Ruellii recta or repens Ruellii
Spanish   Italian   French
German   Dutch

No 30

Plate 117.

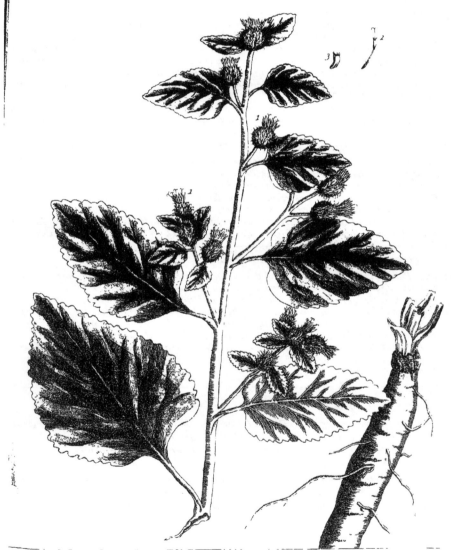

The great Burdock

Fe Black Wither culp et Pinx

1 Flower
2 Flower separate
3 Seed

Bardana major
Lappa major

Plate 118

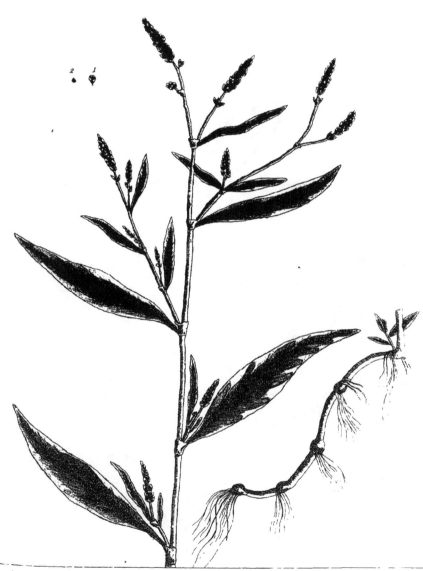

Dead or spotted Arsmart

Fl. Blackwell delin. sculp et Pinx

} 1 Flower
} 2 Seed

{ Persicaria maculata or maculosa

Plate 110.

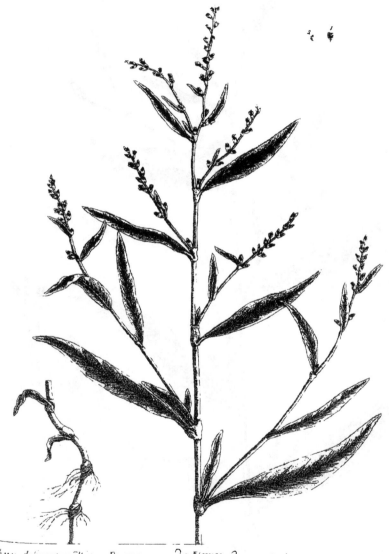

Sharp Smart or Water Pepper   { 1 Flower {   Hydropiper
                              { 2 Seed {

Plate 121

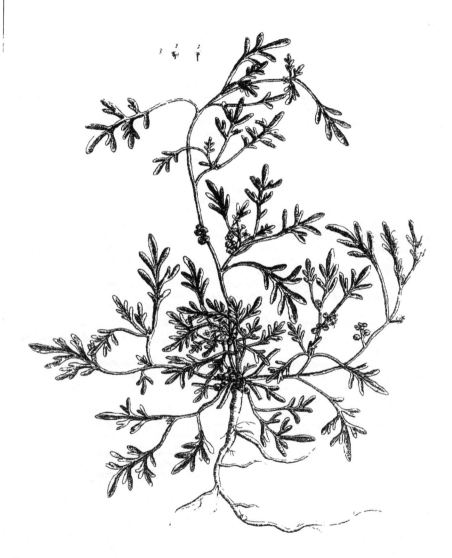

Buckshorn or Swines Cresses {1 Flower} Coronopus Ruellii.
Elaz Blain all dáten ach et Plas. {2 Fruit}
{3 Seed}

Plate 121 The Cornel Tree. Cornus mas

1. This Tree grows to the Size of a Cherry Tree, the Leaves are a deep Green, the Flowers Yellow and the Berries red

2. It grows in Gardens & flowers in March & April, but y Fruit is not ripe till August or September

3. The Fruit is esteem'd cooling drying and binding. Strengthening y Stomach stopping all kinds of Fluxes & Loosness. & is good in Fevers especially if attended with a Diarrhea The Officinal Preparation is the Rob de Cornis

4. Greek, Κραvία Latin, Cornus, and Cornus hortensis mas Spanish Cornizolos Italian, Corniolo. French Cornier German Cornelbaum Dutch Cornoelye

---

Plate 122. Garden Clary Horminum hortense. Sclarea.

1. It grows to be two Foot high: the Leaves are a dull Green on the Face, and hoary on the Backside, the Flowers are a light Blue

2. It grows in Gardens, flowring in June and July

3. Clary is esteem'd warming & drying - Infused in Wine it comforts a cold windy Stomach. Some commend it as a great strengthener of the Reins, helping the Fluor Albus & invigorating a Cold relax'd Womb - Matthiolus recommends y Leaves infused in Vinegar. & a little Honey as good for Boils - The same Author says that the Women in Italy put a single seed into their Eyes when they are troubled with any Redness, humors or Dimness, but Mr Miller gives this Vertue to the Wild Clary

4. Greek Όριvον Latin Horminum hortense and Sclarea Spanish.   Italian Scarleggia French. Orval or Toulebonne German Scharlach Dutch Scarlen

---

Plate 123 Garden Spurge. or Lathyris Cataputia minor & Lathyris .

1. The stalks grow to be three or four Foot high, the Leaves are a bluish Green and the Flowers yellowish

2. It grows in Gardens and flowers for several Months in the Summer

3. Some use this Plant to purge watery Humors, which it does with great Violence both upwards and downwards and is seldome used for this but by Empericks The Milk of the stalks destroy Warts by anointing them with it

- Greek Λαθύρις Latin Lathyris, & Cataputia minor Spanish. Tartago Italian Cataputia minore French Espurge German. Springeraut Dutch. Springskruyd Spurge

---

Plate 124 Shepherd's Staff. Virga Pastoris

1. It grows to be four or five Foot high the Leaves are a light Grass Green and the Flowers yellowish

2. It grows in Marshey Grounds, particularly behind the Bishop of London's House at Fulham.

3. Matthiolus says this has the same Vertues as the Teasels. & y Root of this boiled to the Consistence of Beese Wax in Wine, and kept in a Brazen Vessel is good for a Fistula and Clefts in the Fundament - The Rain Water found in y Hollow of the Leaves is commended by some to cool Inflammations of y Eyes, & to render the Face fair

4. Greek   Latin Virga Pastoris Spanish   Italian Virga di Pastore French Vierge de Pasteur German   Dutch,

Plate 121

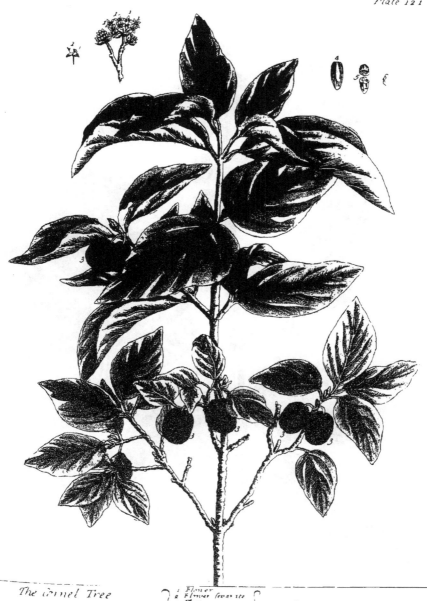

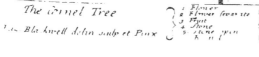

	1 Flower
	2 Flower separate
	3 Fruit
	4 Stone
	5 Stone open

Eliz. Blackwell delin sculp et Pinx   Cornus - mas

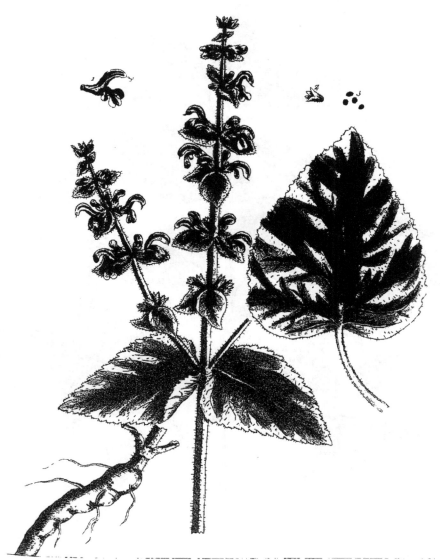

Plate 122

Garden clary

Elis Blackwell delin sculp et Pinx

1. Flower
2. Fruit
3. Seed

terminum hortense Silarea

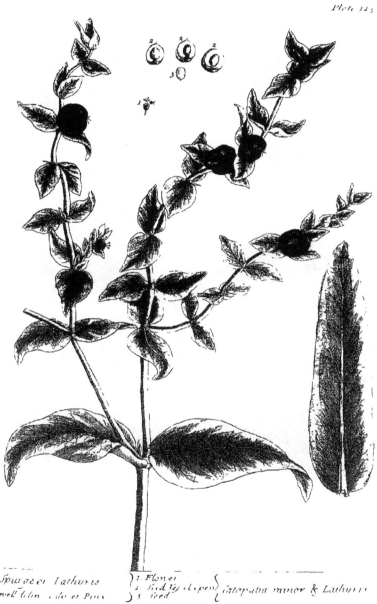

Plate 125

Garden Spurge or Lathuris
Fhe Blackwell delin. ado et Pinx

} 1. Flower
2. Seed Vessel open
3. Seed

Catapatia minor & Lathuris

Plate 121

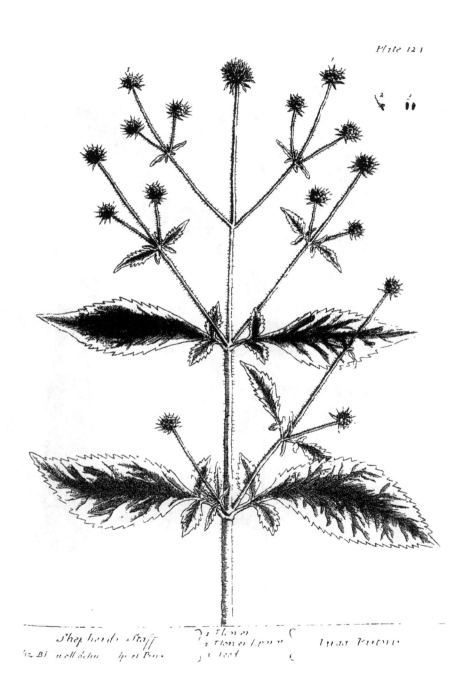

Shepherds Staff

Plate 125 The Fig Tree Ficus

1 It seldome grows to be a Tree of any great Bigness in England, the Leaves are a grass Green and the Fruit when ripe of a brownish Green it beareth no visible Flowers which makes it believed they are hid in the Fruit

2 Its Native soils are Turky, Spain and Portugal, and its time of Bearing is in Spring and Autumn, the Figs are cured by dipping them in scalding hot Lye made of ÿ Ashes of the Cuttings of the Tree and afterwards they dry them carefully in the Sun

3 Figs are esteem'd cooling and moystning, good for Coughs, shortness of Breath and all Diseases of the Breast, as also the Stone and Gravel, and the small Pox and Measels which they drive out - Outwardly they are dissolving and ripening good for Imposthumations and Swellings and pestilential Butoes

4 Greek Σύκα Latin Ficus Spanish. Igos Italian, Fichi French Figues German, Fengen Dutch Uÿoen

---

Plate 126 The Mulberry Tree Morus - mora vulgaris

1 This grows to be a tall Tree, the Leaves are a dark Green the Flowers yellowish and the Berries when ripe a dark Purple

2 It grows in Gardens and the Fruit is ripe in August and September

3 The Bark of the Root is thought to warm and dry, opening obstructions of the Liver and Spleen, and helping the Jaundice - The unripe Fruit is binding and drying, good in all kinds of Fluxes and Inflammations of the Mouth and Throat - The ripe Fruit is cooling, good to allay the Heat of Burning Fevers and create an Appetite

4 Greek. Moéα ἡ συκάμινᵒ Latin, Morus, & Morus arbor Spanish Moras del Moral Italian, Moro French. Maurier German, Maulbeerbaum Dutch Moerbesien

---

Plate 127 The Male Cypress Tree Cupressus mas

1 This grows to be a tall Tree, but is not so much branch'd as the Female the Leaves are a grass Green. the Flowers a dirty Yellow & the Cones which are rounder than ÿ Females brown

2 It grows wild in Creet the Flowers come forth the Beginning of Summer and ÿ Cones are ripe in Autumn

3 The Cones are accounted drying and binding good to stop spitting of Blood, Dyarrheas, Dysenteries, immoderate Flux of the Menses, involuntary Miction They likewise prevent the Bleeding of the Gums and fasten loose Teeth - Outwardly they are used in siptic Fomentations and Cataplasms

4 Greek Κυπάριαος Latin Cupressus mas Spanish. Cipres Italian, Cipresso French, Cypres German, Cipressen Dutch Cypresse Boom

---

Plate 128 Horse Tongue or Double Tongue Hippoglossum Bislingua

1 The Stalks grow five or Six Inches high the Leaves are a deep Green the Flowers whitish. and the Berrys red

2 It grows wild in Italy and flowers in June

3 This Plant is esteem'd heating and drying good for Disorders and Suffocations of the Womb Hysteric Fits, hastening the Birth, expelling the After Birth, and procuring the Catamenia

4 Greek Ἱπποόγλωσον Latin, Bislingua Hippoglossum Spanish Lengua de Cavallo Italian, Bislingua or Bonifacia French Bislingua German Xapfflin craut Dutch

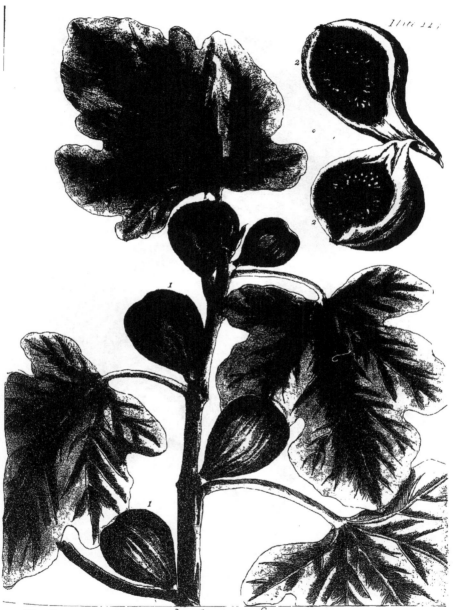

Plate 127

The Fig 1
The Bud knotted in outer 1 Pmk   1 Fruit
2 Fruit op   Fatte

Plate 126

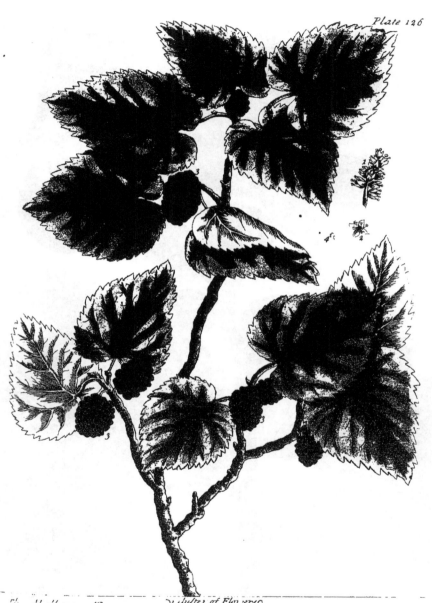

The Mulberry Tree   1 a cluster of Flowers   Morus - mori vulgaris
E. Blackw. fe.   2 a Flower separate
                              3 Fruit

Plate 127

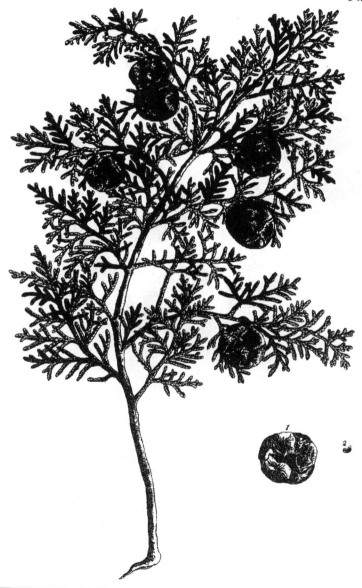

The Male Cypress Tree
Eliz: Blackwell delin. sculp. et Pinx.

} 1 Cone }
} 2 Seed {

Cupressus mas

Plate 118

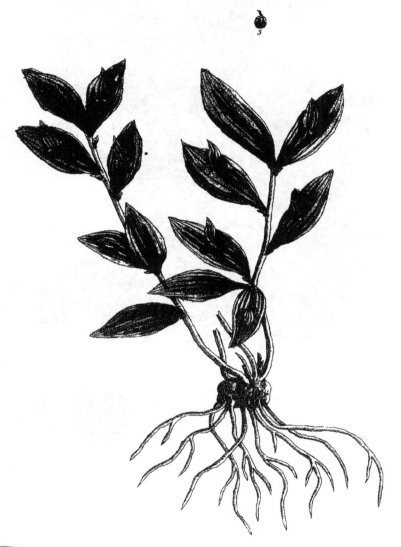

Horse Tongue or Double Tongue 1 Flower ⎰ Hippoglossum Belinova
Eliz Blackwell delin. sculp. et Pinx 2 Berry
3 Berry separate

Plate 129 *Guinea Pepper Capsicum Piper indicum*

The Stalks grow to be two Foot high, the Leaves are a deep grass Green the Flowers white and the Fruit red

1 It is sown in Gardens, and flowers in August the fruit being ripe in September

2 Some commend a Decoction of this with Penny Royal as good to expell a Dead Child The Skins boild and used as a Gargle help the Tooth Ach A Cataplasm of the Seeds powder'd and mixt with Honey applyed to the Throat, is good for the Quinsey It is much used as a Sauce for any Thing that is flatulent and Windy

3 Greek Καψικὸν Latin, Capsicum Siliquastrum Spanish, Pimiento cornuto Italian Pepe d'India French. Poyvre d'Inde German. Indianisch Pfeffer Dutch

---

Plate 130 *Smooth Sow-thistle. Sonchus laevis*

1 It grows about two Foot high, the Leaves are a light grass Green, and the Flowers yellow

2 It grows upon Banks and Way sides, and flowers in May and Iune

3 The Leaves are much of the Nature of Dandelyon, being apperative and diuretic good for the Gravel and Stoppage of Urine Some boil the Leaves in Posset-drink & give it in Fevers The Young Shoots are often eat among Sallads as Lettice

4 Greek Σόγχος Latin, Sonchus laevis Spanish, Serraya Italian Cicerbita French, Laiteron german, Ganddistel Dutch.

Plate 131 *Water Calamint Calamentha aquatica*

1 It grows to be a Foot high, the Leaves are a dull Green, and the Flowers purple

2 It grows in moist Places where Water has stagnated all the Winter and flowers in Iune and Iuly

3 It is hot and dry and is peculiarty appropriated to the female Sex it is esteemd a good Uterine, provoking the Menses and Lochia It warms the Bowels and helps the Cholic and Iaundice

4 Greek Καλαμίνθα ἐνώδης Latin, Calamentha aquatica Spanish Nevedo Italian calamento aquatica French Pouliot de   German Bassermunk Dutch Water calamenth

---

Plate 132 *Groundsel Erigeron Senecio*

1 The Stalks grow to be a Foot high, the Leaves are a light Green and the Flowers yellow

2 It grows on Banks Walls and Rubbish flowering the greatest part of the Year

3 Some take the Iuice of this Herb in Ale as a Gentle Vomit, to ease the Pains in the Stomach evacuate Choler help the Iaundice and destroy Worms Outwardly it is usefull in scrophulous Tumours, and Inflammations of the Breast, and helps scald Heads

4 Greek ήριγέρων Latin Erigeron Spanish Bon varron Italian Cardoncello French Senesson german Creuknurt Dutch Kruiskruyd

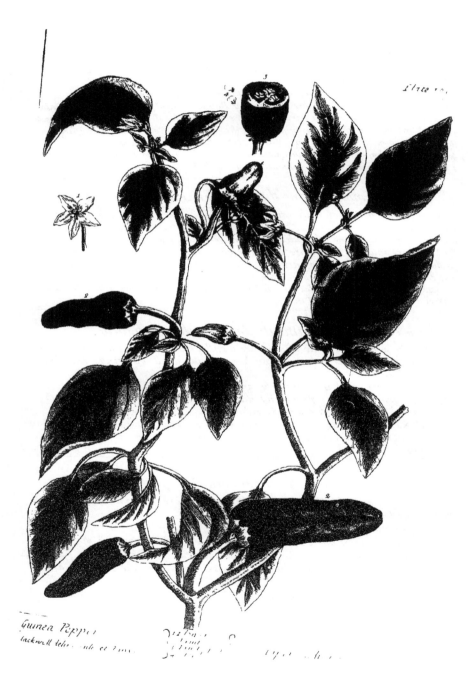

Guinea Pepper
lackwell delin: sulp et Pinx:

Plate 130

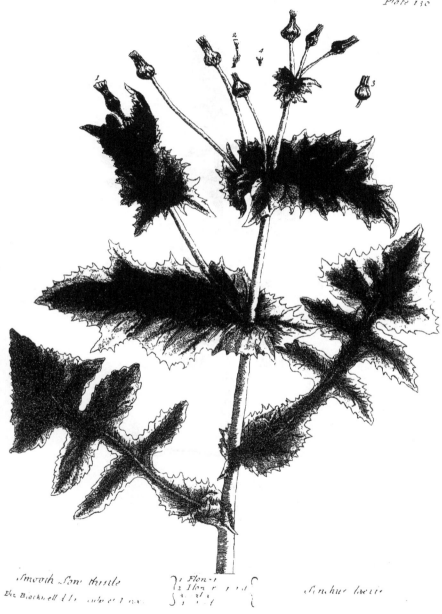

Smooth Sow thistle

Eliz Blackwell d.l. sculp et Pinx.

1 Flow
2 Flow
3 Seed

Sonchus laevis

Plate 15

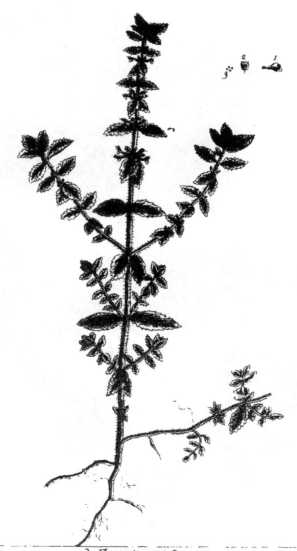

Water Calamint

Eliz: Blackwell delin: sculp: et Pinx:

1 Flower Separate
2 Calix
3 Seed

Calamintha aquatica

Plate 132

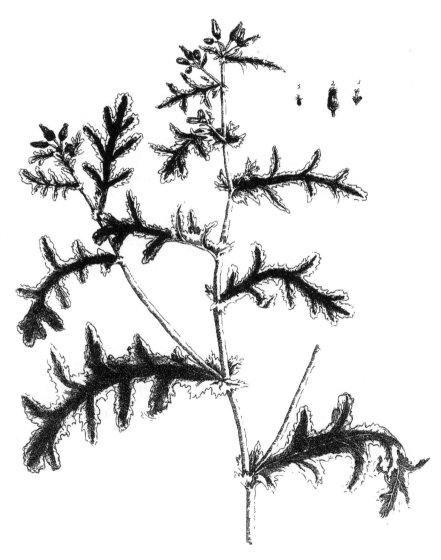

Groundsel

The Burthen

Sorrow parts

2 cals

Erigeron ferens

Plate 133 Love Apple Amoris Pomum

1 The Stalks grow to be two Foot high the Leaves are a light yellowish green and the Flowers yellow

2 It is sowen in Gardens, and flowers in Iuly, the Fruit being ripe in September

3 Love Apple outwardly applyed is esteemed cooling and moystning good for Inflammations, Erusipelas the Iuice is commended in hot Destructions of Rheum upon the Eyes In Italy they eat them with Oil and Vinegar as we do Cucumbers

4 Greek Στρυχνον κηπαῖος Latin Pomum Amoris Solanum pomiferum Spanish Italian, Pomo d Oro French Pomme d Amours German Gold apffell Dutch

---

Plate 134 Mastich Time or Herb Mastich Marum vulgare

It grows to be a Foot high the Leaves are a deep green and the Flowers white

1 It is planted in Gardens, and flowers in Iune and Iuly

2 It is much of the Nature of Marioram some commend it for the too great Flux of the Catamenia a Drachm of the Powder being given in rough Wine Dioscorides commends a Decoction of the Leaves as good for the Dropsy, when it has not got too great a Head and the Leaves mixt with Honey as good for removing the Blackness of any Bruise

3 Greek Σάμψυκον κ̣ Ἁμάρακος Latin, Marum vulgare, Sampsuchus Spanish Mayorana Italian Majorana gentile French, Marone gentil German, Megeran Dutch Mastick ruykende Marum

---

Plate 135 Buckthorn Rhamnus catharticus Spina cervina

1 This Bush has Branches full of long stiff Thorns the Leaves are a yellowish Green, and the Flowers yellow

2 It grows in Woods & Hedges flowers in Iune, and the Berries are ripe in September

3 The Iuice of the Berries purges serous watery Humours, and is esteem'd good for the Gout Dropsy Iaundice Scurvy Itch and all manner of Eruptions in the Skin The Officinal Preparation is the Surupus e Spina Cervina

4 Greek Ῥάμνος Latin Rhamnus catharticus Spina cervina Spanish Scambrones Italian Spino merlo or Spino cervino French Bourgepine ou Nepran German Begdorn, Dutch Rhynbesien

---

Plate 136 Black or Stinking Horehound Marrubium nigrum Ballote

1 The Stalks grow to be two Foot high the Leaves are a dark green and the Flowers a blue Purple

2 It grows by High Ways and Hedges flowering for several Months in the Summer

3 Dioscorides says the Leaves beaten with Salt and applyed to the Wound cures the Bite of a Mad Dog and the Iuice mixt with Honey is good to cleanse foul Ulcers. Doctor Bowle commends it as a singular Remedy against histerical & Hypochondria Affection

4 Greek Βάλλω τῂ Latin Marrubium nigrum or Ballote Spanish Marine negro Italian Marrobio lazzardo French Marrulen noir german Schwartz Andorn Dutch Senart Andooren

No 34

Plate 133

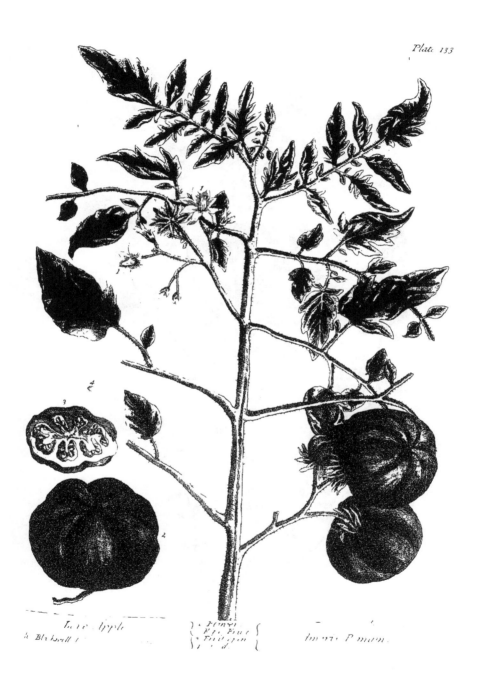

Love Apple
a Blackwell
{ 1 Flower
{ 2 Ripe Fruit
{ 3 Fruit open
Amoris Pomum

Plate 134

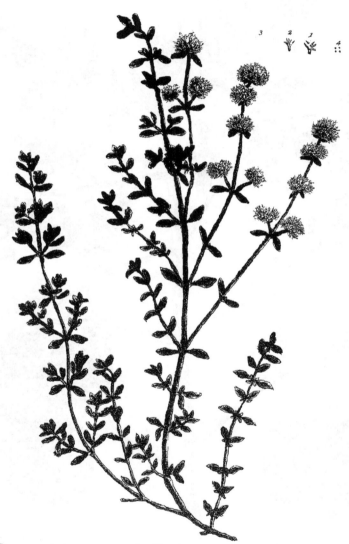

Mastich Time or Herb Mastich

— Blackwell f.

1 Flower
2 ...
3 Flower open
4 seed

Marum colour

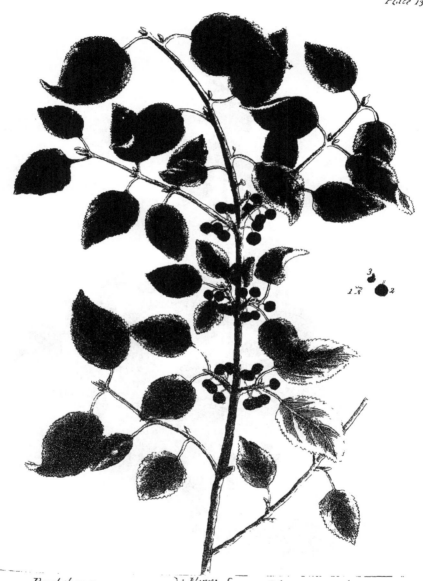

Plate 135

Buckthorn

Eliz Blackwell delin sculp et Pinx

1 Flower
2 Berry
3 Seed

Rhamnus cathartica
Spina cervina

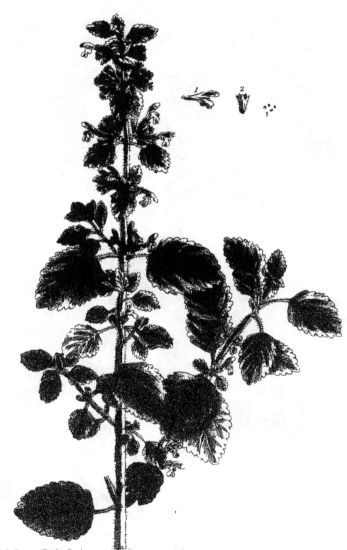

Plate 190

Black or Stinking Horehound

Eliz Blackwell delin sculp et Pinx.

1 Flower separate
2 calex
3 seed

Marrubium nigrum Ballote

Plate 137 *Quinces Cydonea or Mala cotonea majora*

1 This Tree seldom grows so big as the apple Tree, having usually a crooked Body with many weak Branches The Leaves are like those of the apple Tree, but rounder and whitish underneath the Blossomes are a whitish Purple, and the Fruit a yellow Green covered with a Down

2 It is commonly planted by Ponds and Moats, flowring in May, the Fruit being ripe in September and October

3 The Fruit is accounted cordial and strengthning to the Stomach, helping Degestion, and stopping Vomiting & the Hiccough They are also esteemed good for all sorts of Fluxes. The Seed is balsamic and mollifying tempering the Acrimony of Humors & serviceable against sore Mouths Throats, and a Thrush, for which a Mucilage made of them is frequently prescribed Outwardly it is applied to heal sore chopd Nipples

4 Greek Σρθ θιομηλα Latin Cydonea or Cotonea majora Spanish, Membrilhos Italian, Mele cotogne French Pomés de Coing German, Gros Quitten Dutch Quee Boom

---

Plate 138 *Harts Tongue Lingua Cervina, & Phyllitis*

1 This Plant grows to be a Foot high the Leaves are a fine grass Green, the Seed grows in broad oblique Lines on the Backside of the Leaves

2 It grows in Shady Lanes and old Stone Buildings, being green all the Year

3 It is much commended for Disorders of the Liver and Spleen, being good to Dissolve hard schirrhous Tumours in either It is usefull in the Rickets, Spitting of Blood and the Bloody Flux Mr Ray recommends the Powder, or Conserve of y green Leaves, for Histeric & Convulsive Fits, and the Palpitation of the Heart

4 Greek Φυλλιτις Latin, Lingua Cervina Spanish, Lingua cervina Italian Lingua cervina French Lang de Cerf German Hirschtungen Dutch Herts Tonge

---

Plate 139 *Agnus castus, or The Chaste Tree Vitex or Agnus castus*

1 This Tree grows about the Bigness of a small Cherry Tree, the Leaves are a dark green above and whitish underneath the Flowers are a whitish Purple & y Seed a blukish Grey

2 It is a Native of Italy & is planted here in gardens flowring the latter End of Summer

3 The Leaves Flowers & Seed are esteemed warming and drying helps the ardness of the Liver & Spleen expells Wind & brings down y catamenia som rly y Seed was much used to allay venereal heus & preserve chastity but this Age has left that Medicine out of their Dispensatory as useless

4 Greek Αγ s και λ y os Latin Vitex Agnus castus Felix nenerina Spanish Gattiglio casto Italian Vitice or Vino casto French casto German Schafmudet Dutch Kuis Boom

---

Plate 140 *Privet or prim Print Ligustrum*

1 This is a low Shrub the Leaves are a grass green the Flowers white & the Berries Black

2 It grows in Hedges and flowers in May & June y Berries being ripe in September

3 The Leaves and Flowers are accounted cold and drying & astringent good for Ulcers & Inflammations of y Throat Bleeding of the Gums and Relaxation of the Uvula Dioscorides commends the Flowers steepd in Vinegar as good for the Head ach

4 Greek Κυπρος Latin Ligustrum Spanish Alfena or Sallena Italian Guistrico Olivella French Troesne or Trezillon German Beinholtz oder Dutch Mondhout keelkruyd

No 35

Plate 137

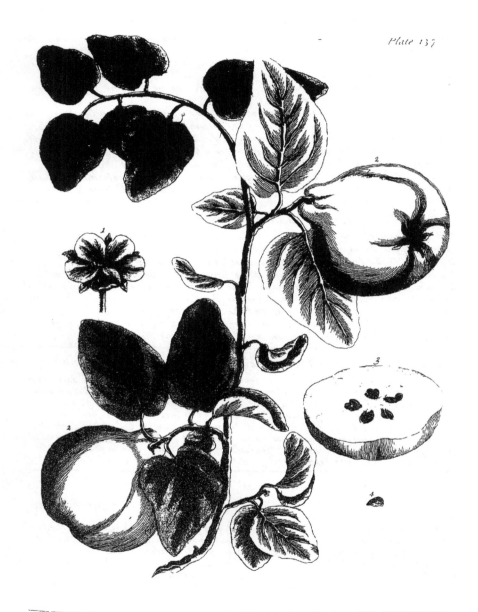

Quince
Eliz Blackwell delin: sculp et Pinx

Blossome
Fruit

cydonia
a Mala cotonea majora

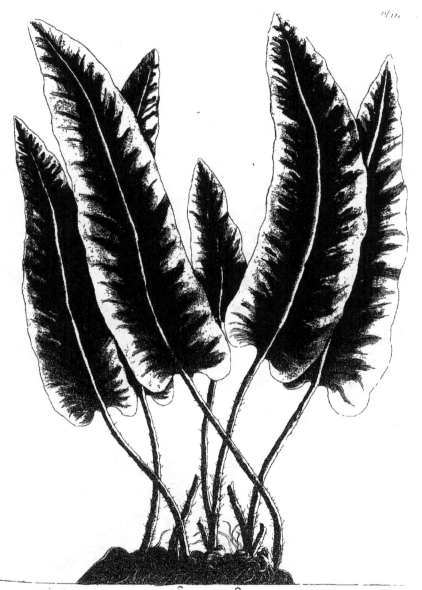

Scolop. Lingua

the Broad Hollow tongue Prax

Lingua cervino
{ ...ud. }

Lingua cervino
d'India

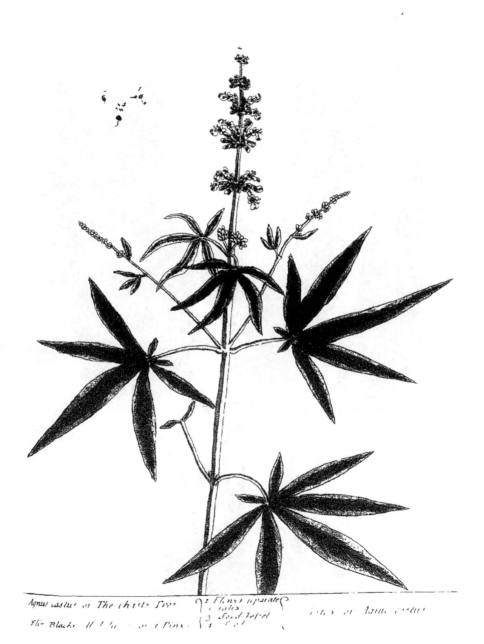

Agnus castus or The chaste Tree   1 Flower separated
                                   2 Calix
Flos Blacks   3 Seed Vessel   ... of Agnus castus
                                   4 Seed

Plate 140

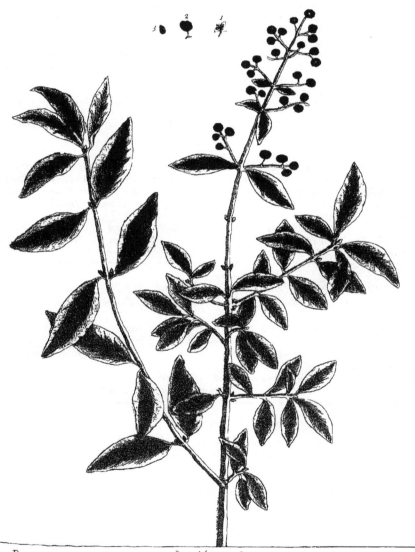

Privet or prim Print

I'iz Blacknell delin catfiet Priv

) 1 flower (
(2 berry (
(3 ? ( )

Ligustrum

Plate 141 The Apple Tree Malus sativa

1. Among the great variety of Apples, those which are accounted best or Medicinal Use are the Pearmain and Pippin - The largest Pearmain is here in Herefordshire The Leaves are a dark grass Green above, and hoary underneath and the Blossoms white tinctured with purple
2. It is planted in Gardens and flowers in March
3. Apples are accounted cordial, chearing the Spirits and driving away Melancholy of the Juice is made the Syrup of Pomes, which is an Ingredient in ye Confectio Alkermes
4. Greek Mηλέα Latin, Malus sativa Spanish Mansanas Italian, Mele, or Pome French, Pomes German Depfell   Dutch Appelen

---

Plate 142 Devils Bit, or smooth Succisa Morsus Diaboli & Succisa

1. The Stalks grow to be a Foot and a half high, the Leaves are a grass green and the Flowers a blue Purple
2. It grows in Meadows and Pasture Grounds and flowers ye latter end of Summer
3. The Leaves are esteem'd alexipharmic useful in malignant Fevers and Pestilential Distempers Outwardly as a Cataplasm they are good for Bruises and Contusions The Herb Women sell the Leaves of this Plant instead of the common Scabious
4. Greek   Latin Succisa or Morsus Diaboli Spanish Italian, Morso di Diavolo French   German Zeuffels Abbiss Dutch Duvvels Beed

---

Plate 143 Male Speedwell Veronica mas

1. This is a low creeping Plant the Leaves are a light Green and the Flowers a bluish Purple
2. It grows in Woods and Shady Places, flowring in June
3. This is esteemed a vulnerary Plant being used both inwardly & outwardly Some account it good for coughs and consumptions the Stone Stranguary and pestilential Fevers
4. Greek   Latin Veronica mas Spanish   Italian Veronica French   German Ehrenpreis Dutch

---

Plate 144 Saffron Crocus

1. The Stalks grow four or five Inches above ground The Leaves are a dark grass Green, and the Flowers purple, with red Stamina which is ye Saffron of the Shops
2. The best saffron grows in Essex Suffolk and Cambridgeshire it flowers in September and October
3. Saffron is esteemed a great cordial strengthening ye heart & usual parts resisting Putrefaction & usefull in all kinds of malignant & Contagious Distempers Fevers small Pox & Measles It opens obstructions of ye Liver & Spleen help's ye Jaundice brings down ye Catamenia expediates the Birth & expells ye Secundines It is also good in Diseases of ye Lungs as Asthmas or consumptions Outwardly in Poultices eases Pain & ripens Imposthums
4. Greek, Κρόκος Latin Crocus & Crocus sativus Spanish Izafran Italian Zaffarano French Zaffran German Saffran Dutch Saffraan

No 30

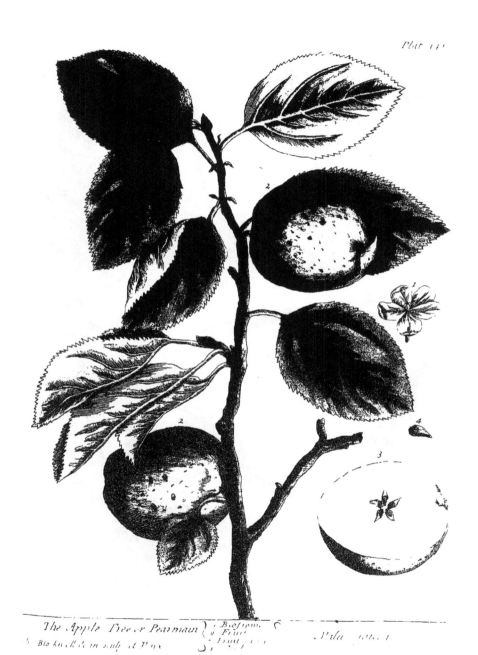

The Apple Tree or Pearmain } 1 Blossom.
2 Fruit
3 Fruit

Blackwell delin sculp et Pinx

N° 141

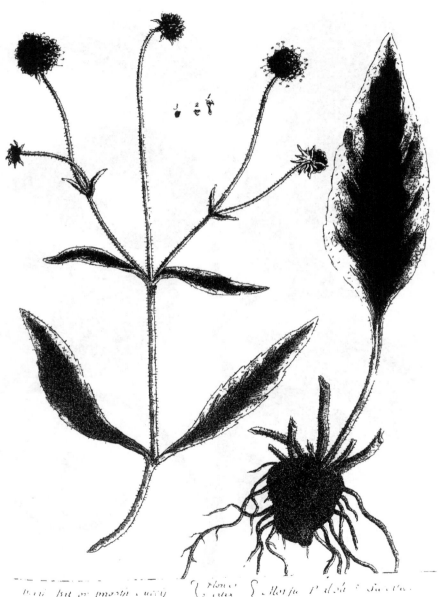

Plate 143

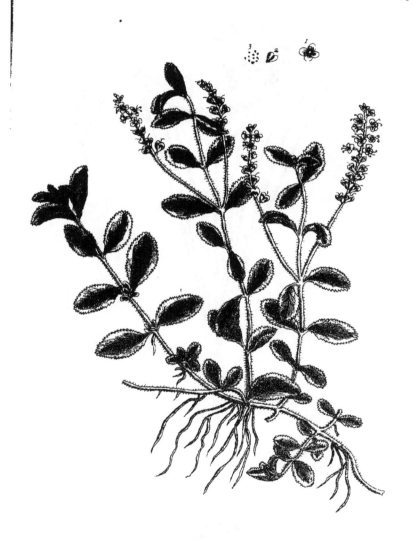

Male Speedwell
Bl. Blackwell del. sculp. et Pinx.

1 Flower.
2 Seed Vessell.
3 Seed

Veronica mas

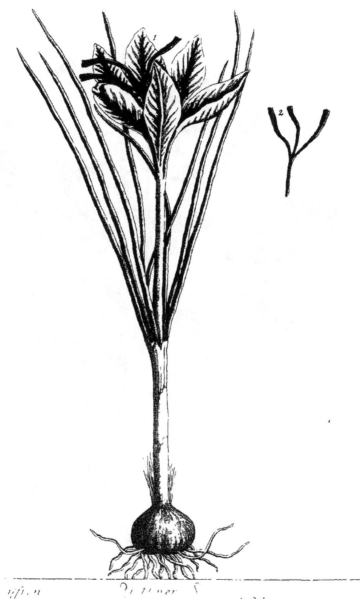

Plate 145 *Pomgranates* Granata, Punica mala

The Pomgranate Tree which bears Fruit produces a single Flower of the same colour as the double, and the Tree it self differs very little from the other

1 This Tree as well as the other, grows in Spain Italy and the warm countries

2 The single Flowers are drying and restringent good for Hemorrhagies & Bleedings both inward and outward The Fruit is gratefull and strengthning to the Stomach stops Looseness and the immoderate Flux of the Terms, and is usefull in hot bilose Fevers, and gonorrheas

3 Greek Póïa Latin Granata Spanish Granadas Italian, Melagrano, or Pomo granato French, Pomes de grenades or Mygrains German, Granatopffelbaum Dutch, Granaat Boom

---

Plate 146 *Tobacco* Petum Tabaccum

1 It grows to be three Foot high, the Leaves are a grass green, & y Flowers a pale Red

2 It is sown in the Spring and flowers in July and August

3 The Green Leaves are used in Ointments and Oils for Wounds Ulcers, Inflammations Tumours Piles and the Kings Evil. The dryed Leaves are a strong Emetic, & ought to be used with great caution - chew'd or smoak'd it evacuates Phlegm - A Drop of the Dystalled oil taken inwardly will kill a Cat sometimes this Oil is dropt into a hollow Tooth to cure the Tooth-Ach The Dust destroys Fleas Lice & other Vermine

4 Greek Yooκίαμος Latin Petum Hyoscyamus Peruvianus Spanish Petun and Tabus Italian French, Herba de la Roine Mere German India mich Bundternut Dutch Taback

---

Plate 147 *Sow-bread* Artanita, cyclamen.

1 The Stalks grow to be six or eight Inches high the Leaves are a grass green spotted with white above & purplish underneath & the Flowers a pale Red

2 It is planted here in Gardens flowring in September and October, its Native Places being the Alps, Austria & Styria

3 The Root is very forcing and usefull to bring away the Birth and Secundines and provoke the Menses Some commend the Juice against vertiginous Disorders of y Head, used in form of an Errhine, it is also good for cutaneous Eruptions

4 Greek Κυκλαμινος Latin Artanita cyclamen Spanish Pan de Puerco Italian Pan Porcino French cyclamen or Pain Porcin German, Schweinbrot Dutch, Darkensbrood

---

Plate 148 *The greater Spurge* or Palma Christi Catapntia mayor & Ricinus

1 The Plant grows to be Six or Seven Foot high, the Leaves are a fine grass green the Flowers are small and staminous of a yellow colour

2 It is planted in Gardens, and flowers late in the Summer

3 The Kernels are used by some to purge watery Humors but they must be used with great Caution The Oil express'd from the Seeds is good to destroy Lice in childrens Heads

4 Greek Κικι ή κροτων Latin, Ricinus Spanish Figueira del Inferno Italian Mirasole French, Palma Christi German Bunderlaum Dutch, Donderboom

No 37

Plate 145

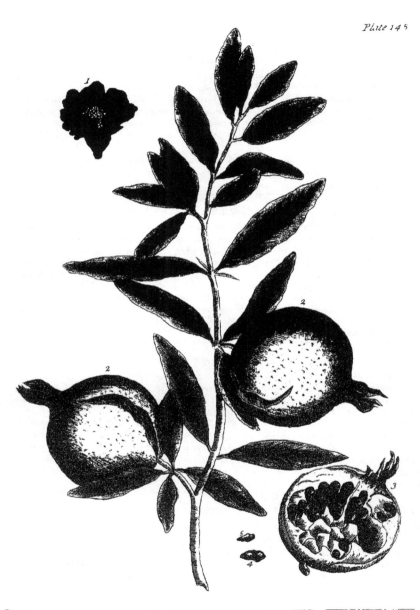

Pomeranates

Faz Blackwell delin. culp et Pinx

1 Flower
2 Fruit
3 Fruit open { Granata Punica mala
4 Bour
5 Seed

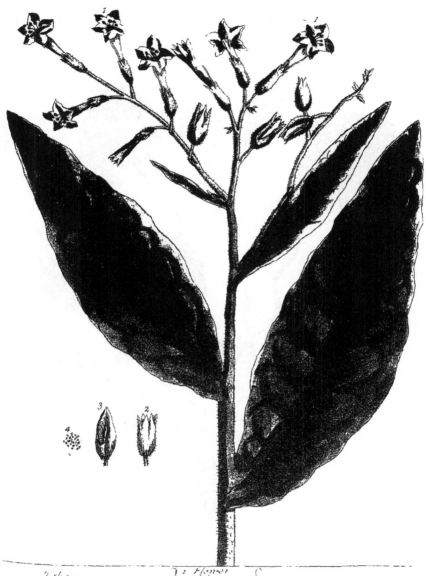

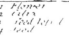

Table 43

Tobacco

1 *Flower*
2 *Calix*
3 *Seed Vessel*
4 *Seed*

Plate 147

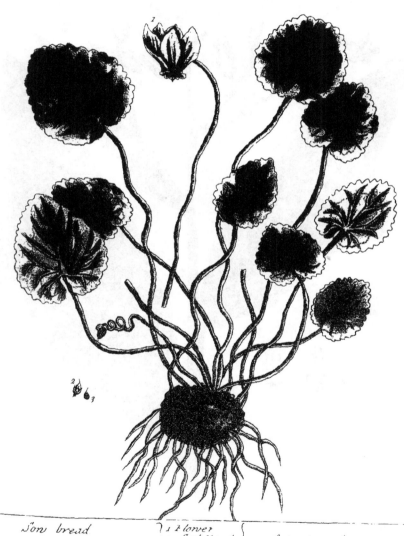

Sow bread

Eliz. Blackwell delin & Pinx

1 Flower
2. Seed Vessel
3. Seed

Artanita Cyclamen

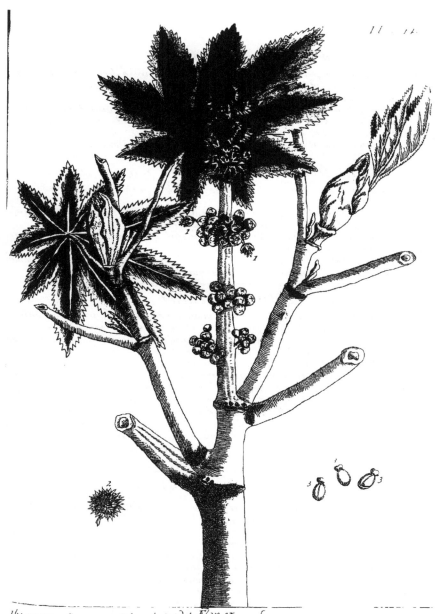

The greater Spurge or Palma christi } 1 Flower

E. Blackwell ...   Ricinus

Plate 149   Haw thorn. Spina Alba

1. This grows to be a pretty large Tree the Leaves are a deep grass Green, the Flowers white with reddish Apices in the Middle and the Berries red

2. It flowers in May, and the Fruit is ripe in September

3. The Flowers & Fruit are both used in the Shops, and are accounted diuretic, good for ÿ Stone, Gravel, & Pleurisy The Aqua Nephritica is made of the Flowers

4. Greek, Μεσπίλος Latin, Mespilus, Oxyacanthus Spanish, Azarolo Italian, Azarolo French, Nesplier German, Dornbaum Dutch, Doornboom

---

Plate 150   Musk Crane's Bill   Geranium moschatum

1. The Stalks grow to be a Foot high, the Leaves are a light grass Green, and the Flowers purple

2. It is generally planted in Gardens, flowring great part of the Summer, some times it is found Wild in several Parts of England

3. This is accounted a vulnerary Plant and is useful in inward Wounds Bruises and Haemorrhages and most Fluxes

4. Greek, Γεράνιον Latin Geranium moschatum Spanish Pico de Cicuenha Italian Geranio terzo French. Bec de Cicongne German. Storchschnabel Dutch

---

Plate 151   Elder   Sambucus

1. This is a common Hedge Tree & seldom grows to any great bigness the Leaves are a light grass Green, the Flowers white, and the Berries a deep purple

2. It grows frequently in Hedges near Ditches and flowers in May the Berries being ripe in September

3. The Bark, Leaves, Flowers & Berries are used. The inner Bark is much used for the Dropsy - The Leaves outwardly are good for Inflammations St Anthony's Fire & the Piles, the Flowers are used for the same, and are also put in Fomentations & Cataplasms for all kinds of Swellings Tumours, & Pains in the Limbs inwardly they expell Wind & help the Cholic The Berries are cordial & useful in hysteric Disorders on the Trunk of this Tree grows an Excrescence which they call Jews Ears being accounted good for ÿ Swelling & Inflammation of the Tonsils, sore Throats and Quinseys

4. Greek, Ακτῆ Latin, Sambucus Spanish, Savinero Italian Sambuco French Suyer German Holder Dutch Vlierboom

---

Plate 152   Black Alder   Alnus nigra

1. This Tree never grows to any great Bigness, the Leaves are a grass Green the Flowers white and the Berries black

2. It grows in moist thick Woods, as Hampstead and Hornsey, and flowers in May the Fruit being ripe in September

3. The Inner Bark purges serous Humours and is commended for ÿ Dropsy & Jaundice but it ought to be prepared with proper aromaticks or else it will cause griping and Vomiting beaten in a Mortar and mixd with Vinegar it is counted good for the Itch the Parts being washd with the expressd Liquor

4. Greek, Πλάταγα μέλας Latin Alnus nigra, and Frangula Spanish Italian Frangula French Aune noir German Faulbaum Dutch Pulhout Sporkenboom

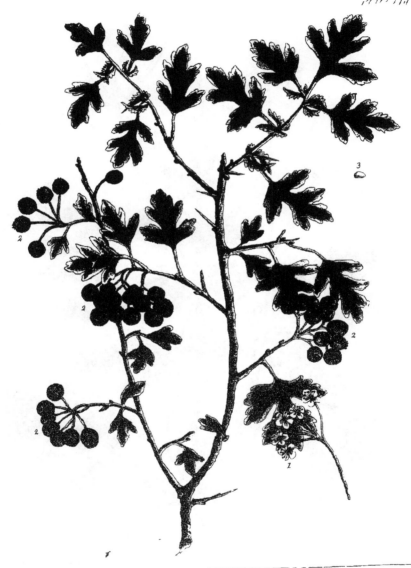

Plate 149

3

2

2

2

2

1

Haw thorn   1 Flower   Spina alba

F. Blackwell f. t.   .   1 Pina   2 Fruit

3 Stone

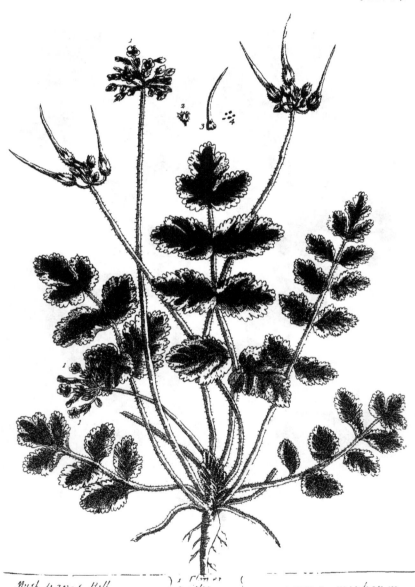

Plate 170

Musk Crane's Bill

½ Blackwell delin. ¼ nat.   1 Flower   Geranium moschatum
                            2 Seed vessel

Plate 151

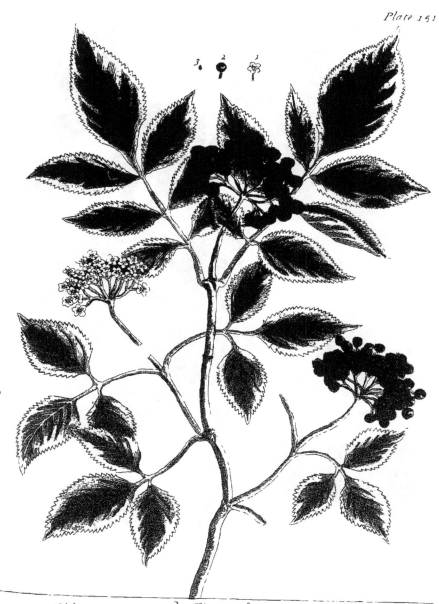

Elder

Eliz Bla kwell delin sculp et Pinx

1. Flower
2 Berry
3 Pod.

Sambucus

Plate 174

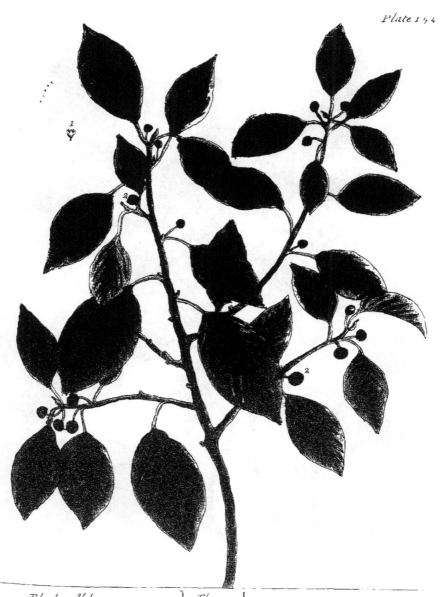

Black Alder   { 1 Flower }   Alnus nigra
Illus L'Admiell del. sculp. ex Pinx { 2 Fruit }

Plate 153 The Vine *Vitis Vinifera*

1. The Vines generally differ according to the Countries they grow in both in Height and Fruit this Vine is the Uvae passae majores or Raisins of the Sun
2. This Vine is a Native of the warm Countries as Spain Portugal Italy and France, it flowers in April and the Grapes are ripe the latter End of Summer
3. Wine is accounted cordial strengthens the Stomach, helps Digestion, comforts y Bowels and is a great Preservative against the Plague. The Raisins of the Sun are made by cutting the Stalks of the Branches when on the Tree almost in two by which means they hinder the sap from coming to them in so great a Quantity as it would do other ways till by the Heat of y Sun & Defect of Nourishment they are sufficiently cured
4. Greek Αμπελος οινοφορος Latin, Vitis, Vinifera Spanish Italian, Vite Vinifera French Vigne German Weinreb Dutch,

Plate 154 The Medlar Tree *Mespilus*

1. It grows as big as an Apple Tree the Leaves are a grass Green the Flowers white, and the Fruit when ripe of a brownish Green
2. It is planted in Gardens flowers in May and the Fruit is ripe in November
3. Medlars are esteem'd cooling drying and binding (especially before they are quite ripe) and are useful in all Kinds of Fluxes Some commend the Hard Seed as good for y Gravel and Stone They are an Ingredient in the Syrupus Mirtinus
4. Greek Μεσπιλος, η μεσπιλη Latin. Mespilus sativa Spanish, Nesper Italian. Nespolo French Nesplier German Nespel Dutch

Plate 155 Kneeholm or Butcher's-broom *Bruscus or Ruscus*

1. The Stalks grow to be a Foot high, the Leaves are a deep Green, the Flowers yellow with a purple Umbel in the Middle and the Berries red
2. It grows in Hedges and Thickets, particularly on Epping Forrest, and flowers for several Months in the Summer
3. The Root is one of the five opening Roots, and is accounted good for Obstructions of the Liver and Spleen, the Jaundice and Dropsy It is a strong Diuretic provokes Urine helps the Gravel and Stone, and brings down the catamenia Tournefort commends a Conserve of the Berries to stop a Gonorrhea
4. Greek Μυοσ ι η αγρια & Οξυμυρσινη Latin Oxymirsine Spanish Jus barba, and Gil barbera Italian, Brusco & Pongitopi French Brus German, Bruch Rensdorn Dutch

Plate 156 Pellitory of the Wall *Parietaria, Helxine*

1. It grows to be Eight Inches high, the Leaves are a dark Green and y Flowers red before they are full blown and white afterwards
2. It grows upon old Walls, and flowers in May
3. The whole Herb is used being cooling opening and cleansing containing a nitrous sulphureous Salt, which recommends it for the Stone Gravel, Stoppage in fort of Urine, for which Ends the Juice or Decoction is given at the Mouth and in Glisters Some commend it for Coughs.
4. Greek Ελξινη η περδικιον Latin Helxine Spanish Yerva del muro Italian Vetriola French Paritoire German Zraunt Richt Dutch

V 30

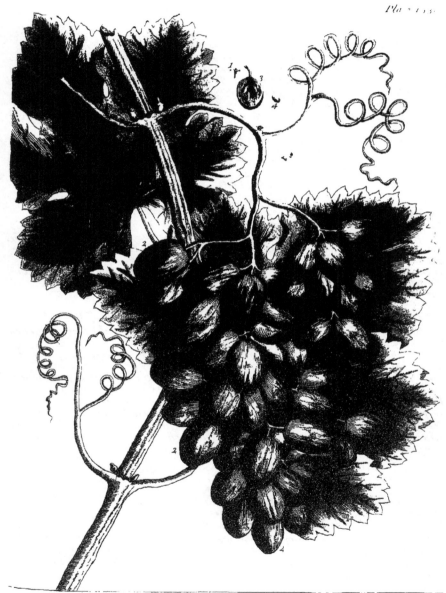

Plate 155

The Vine.

1 Flower
2 Fruit
3 Fruit open
4 ston

I.z Blackwell in sculp. et Pinx.

Vitis vinifera.

Plate 154

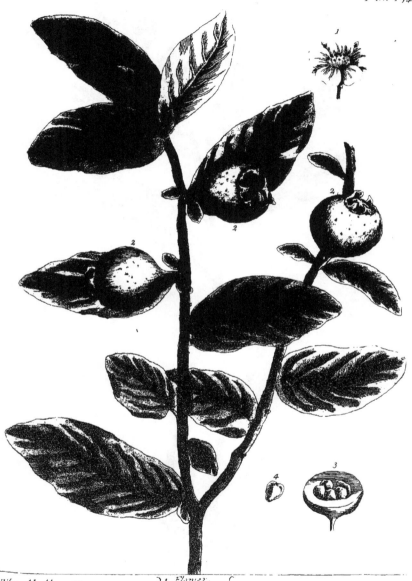

The Medlar Tree

1 Flower.
2 Fruit
3 Fruit cut
4 Seed

Mespilus

Plate 155

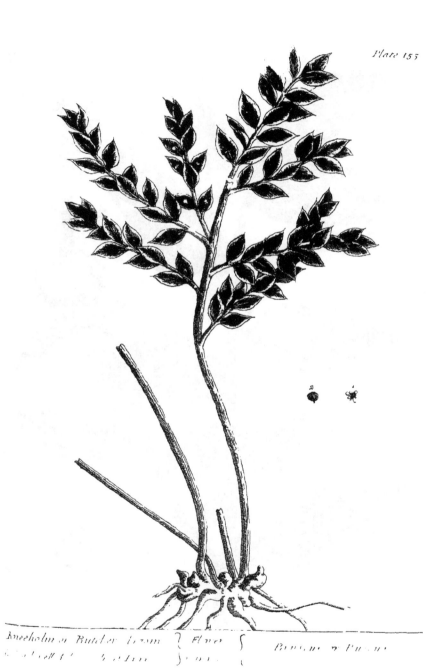

Kneeholm or Butcher broom } Flores { Bruscus m Prusc[...]

Plate 156.

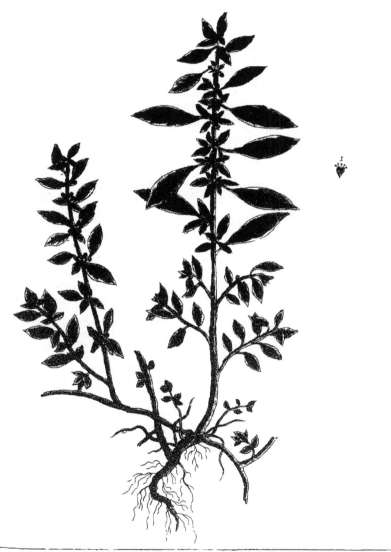

Pellitory of the Wall } 1. Flower { Parietaria Herba

Eliz. Blackwell del. sculp et Pinx

Plate 157 *The Citrul or Water-melon Citrullus or Anguria*

1 The Stalks creep on the ground like the Stalks of a Cucumber the Flowers are yellow and the Fruit Green, and commonly grows as big as a Pomkin

2 It is much cultivated in the Warm Countries as Italy Spain Turkey the East & West Indies, and flowers according to the Months it is sown in

3 Water Melons are much esteem'd for their cooling and refreshing Quality, being very serviceable in great Heats The Seed is one of the greater Cold Seeds and is much of the Nature of Melon and Cucumber agreeing with them in their cooling diuretic Faculties

4 Greek   Latin, Anguria Spanish, Cogombro Italian Anguria French Cocombres German Erdopffel Dutch Cocomero

---

Plate 158 *Wild Iris or Stinking Gladwyn Iris silvestris spatula fœtida*

1 It grows to be a Foot high, the Leaves are a grass Green, and the Flowers a dull Colour with purple Veins, and the Seed Red

2 It grows in Hedges and Thickets, particularly by Jack Straws Castle beyond Islington, and flowers in Iune

3 Some account the Root a Specific for the Kings-Evil, and scrophulous Swellings both given inwardly and applied outwardly It is said also to provoke Urine, and to be usefull in Hysteric Disorders

4 Greek, ξυρις Latin, Xyris Spanish, Lirio Spadanal Italian Spatola fetida French, Glaicul German, Baudtleuscraut Dutch

---

Plate 159 *Rosemary. Rosmarinus*

1 This Shrub grows larger in England than in most Countries, the Leaves are hoary underneath and a dark green above and the Flowers a pale Purple

2 It grows wild in Spain & y Southern Parts of France, but it is planted here in Gardens flowring in April

3 It is accounted good for affections of the Head & Nerves It strengthens y Sight and Memory, and opens Obstructions of the Liver & Spleen - The Dried Herb burnt is good to sweeten the Air Officinal Preparations are, Conserva Anthos, Aqua Reginae Hungariae the Chymical Oil and fixd Salt

4 Greek Λιβανωτις στεφανωματικη Latin Libanotis or Rosmarinum coronarium Spanish, Romero Italian Rosmarino coronario French, Rosmarin German Rosmarin Dutch, Rosemaryn

---

Plate 160 *Flax Linum*

1 The Stalks grow to be a Yard high, the Leaves are a grass Green and the Flowers blue

2 It is sown in Fields and flowers in Iune

3 Linseed is esteem'd emollient digesting and ripening, of great use in Inflammations, Tumours and Imposthumes Cold drawn Linseed Oil is of great Service in all Distempers of the Breast and Lungs - It also helps the Collic and Stone, both taken at the Mouth, and given in Glysters

4 Greek Λινον Latin, Linum sativum Spanish, Lino Italian Lino French Lin German, Lein or Flacks Dutch Vlas

No 40.

Plate 151

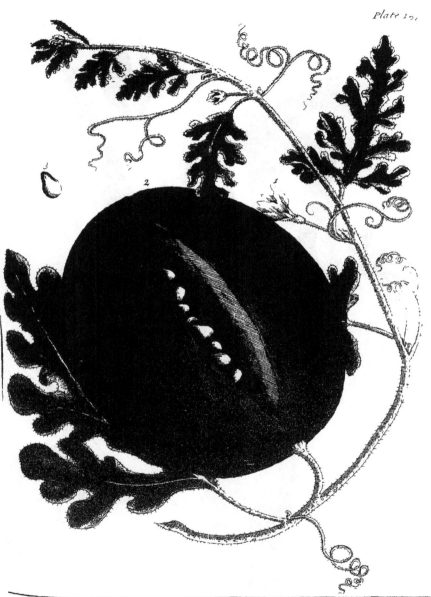

The Gurul or Water-melon   1. Flower   citrullus or tennus
by Blackwell delin sculp et tern.   2. Fruit   3. Seed

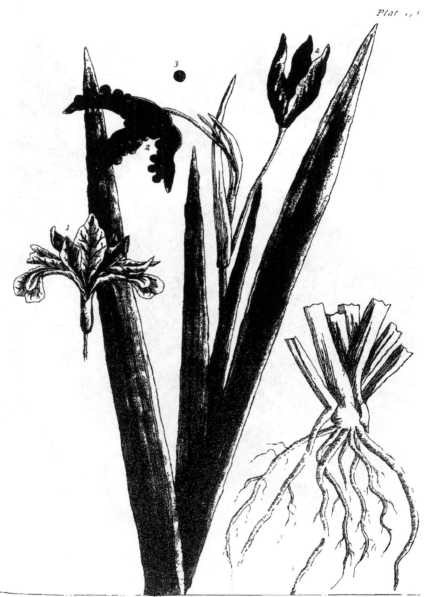

3

Wild Iris or Stinking gladwin {1 Flower} {Iris plustris Spatula fatida
Enz Blackwell dehn ... ej et Pinx {...}

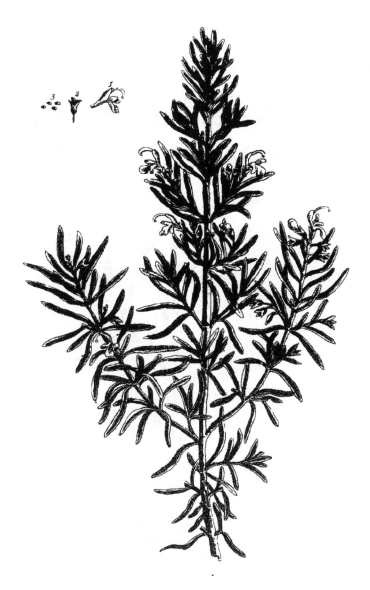

Rosemary
1 Blossell the colon Pan   1 Flowerspread   Rosmarinus
5 Seed

Plate 1

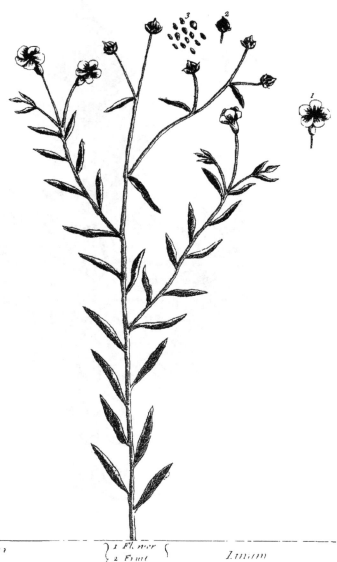

Flax

Linum

1. Flower
2. Fruit
3. Seed

Plate 101 Red Winter cherries Alkekengi or Halicacabum

1. The Stalks grow two Foot high, the Leaves are a dull green the Flowers white with yellow Stamina and the Fruit red
2. They are planted here in gardens flowering in July and August the Fruit being ripe in September
3. The Leaves are esteem'd cooling, and the Berries a good Diuretic usefull in the Gravel and Stone - Boiled in Milk and sweetned with Sugar they cure the Heat of Urine making bloody Water Ulcers in the Kidneys and Bladder They help the Jaundice by opening the Obstructions of the Liver and Gall Bladder, and the Dropsy by carrying off the Water thro the Urinary Passages The officinal Preparation is the Trochises Alkekengi
4. Greek Στρυχνος αλικάκαβος Latin Solanum vesicarium Spanish Besaa de Perro Italian Alcachengi French Buguenandes German Judentschen Dutch Krieken van Oberzee

---

Plate 102 French Mercury Mercurialis mas & foemina

1. It grows about a Foot high, the Leaves are a mild green & the Flowers yellowish
2. It grows frequently in Gardens waste Places and Rubbish flowring for several Months in the Year
3. The Leaves and Stalks are accounted apperative and mollifying a Decoction of them purges choleric and serous Humours, used in Clisters - Matthiolus commends a Decoction of the Seed with Wormwood for the yellow Jaundice The Juice is good to take away Warts
4. Greek Λινόζωστις θηλυς Latin Mercurialis vulgaris mas et foemina Spanish Mercuriale Italian Mercurella femina French Mercuriale femelle german Bingelcraut Weible Dutch

---

Plate 103 The smaller Spurge Esula minor Pituusa

1. The Stalks grow more than a Foot high, the Leaves are a grass green and the Flowers yellowish
2. It is planted in gardens here, & flowers for several Months in the Summer
3. This Plant is a violent strong Cathartic & Emetic and is said to be good in the Dropsy Gout, & other Obstinate Distempers But must be used with great Caution
4. Greek Τιθυμαλος χαραγιανια Latin Esula minor Spanish Lecce tirigua Italian Esula minore French Tithumale german Ejpejene Bolffwolfh Dutch

---

Plate 104 Chickweed Usine

1. It grows to be eight Inches high, the Leaves are a light grass green and the Flowers white
2. It grows every where in moist Places and too often in Gardens flowring most Months in the Year
3. It is esteem'd cooling and moistning good for Inflammations of the Liver St Anthonys Fire, Redness and Pimples in the Face being applied to be Part affected as a Cataplasm or Cloths dipt in the Juice and Poultice made of it and helps hot Swellings & Tumours the Juice droped into the Eye helps Redness Pustules
4. Greek Αλσιν Latin Alsine Spanish Indies Pepnine French Mouron german Boschleraut Dutch Muur

No 41

Plate 101

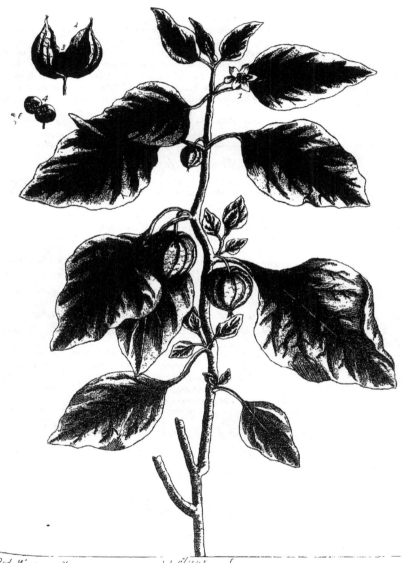

Red Winter Cherries

The Blackwell delin. sculp. et Pinx

Ukekenqu n tuluntalra

Plate 104

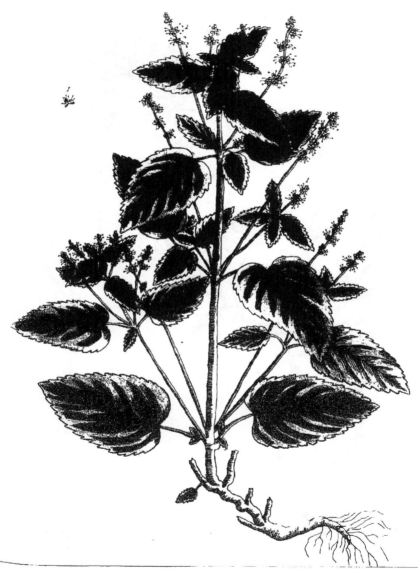

French Mercury

Eliz Bla. knoll delin. culp. et Pinx

{ 1 Flower }

Mercurialis mas & ficmina

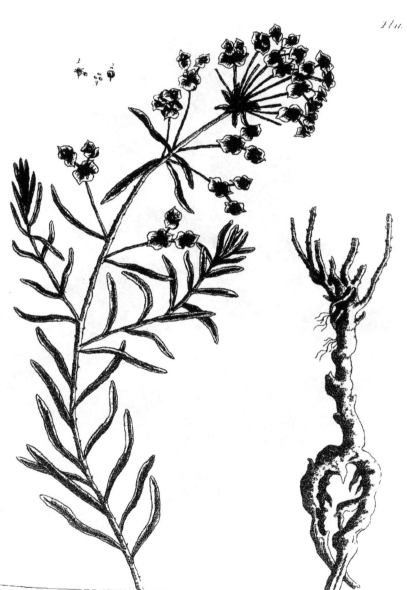

The *smaller* Spurge

2 Blackwell delin: and Pinx:

Esula minor Tithous a

Plate 104

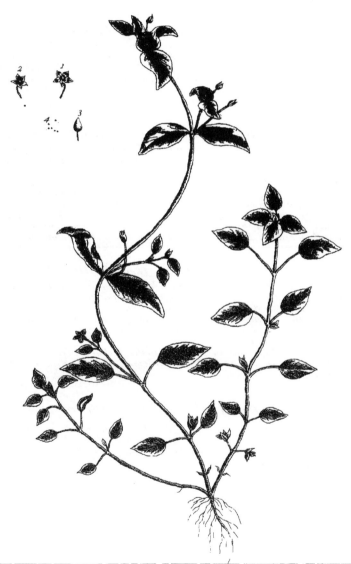

Chickweed

Eliz Blackwell delin. sculp et Pinx

1 Flower
2 Calix
3 Seed Vesel
4 Seed

Flame

Plate 105 The Barberry Bush Berberis Oxyacantha

1 It seldom grows to any great Bigness the Leaves are a fine grass green the Flowers yellow and the Berries red

2 In some Parts they grow wild and are also planted in Gardens, flowering in May, the Berries being ripe in September

3 The Inner Bark of this Bush is accounted a Specific for the Yellow Jaundice either taken in an Infusion or Decoction, being opening and attenuating The Berries are good to moisten the Mouth and quench Thirst in Burning Fevers being cooling & restringent The Conserve is serviceable against all kinds of Loosness Fluxes & ye Jaundice The Seed is esteemd binding & restringent The officinal Preparation is the Conserve of the Fruit

4 Greek Οξυακανθα Latin Oxyacantha Spanish   Italian, Crespino French Vinette German, Bersich Dutch, Barberisse

---

Plate 106 Mountain Calamint Calamentha montana

1 It grows to be a Foot high the Leaves are a deep Green, & ye Flowers a pale Purple

2 There are two sorts of this Calamint found in Kent in great Plenty, growing by Hedges and flowring in June and July

3 This Calamint is hotter than Common Mint being a good Stomatic, expelling Wind, and helping the Collic It is of great Service to the Female Sex, in Obstructions of the Catamenia bringing them to a regular Course this it does taken inwardly or by a strong Decoction given as a Clyster The officinal Preparation is the Pulv Diacal simplex

4 Greek Καλαμινθα ορινη Latin Calamentha vulgaris montana Spanish, Nereda Italian, Nipotella montana French, Poullio montagne german, Bergmuint Dutch Calamenth

---

Plate 107 The Common Calamint, the Shops Calamentha officinalis

1 This Calamint is much like the former only this lyes much upon the Ground and the leaves are smaller the Leaves and Flowers are alike in colour to the former

2 It grows in like Places as the former but flowers in July and August

3 It has much the same Vertues as the other being opening and deobstruent, and is used often for the other, because it grows in greater Plenty and the Shops are mostly supplied with this

4 Greek Καλαμινθα   Latin Calamenthi officinalis n Pulegio etiam Nepeta Spanish Nereda Italian, Calamenta French, Poullio commune german Bilder polen Dutch Berg Calamenth

---

Plate 108 White Ladies-Bed-Straw Gallium album latifolium

1 It grows to be two Foot high, the Leaves are a grass green, and the Flowers White

2 It grows on Banks and dry barren Places flowering in June and July

3 This Plant is esteemd drying and incrassating good to stop all kinds of Fluxes and Haemorrhagies and cure Wounds Some commend a Decoction of it upon the join and a Bath made of it to refresh ye Feet when tired with overmuch walking In the North they use this Plant instead of Rennet in making their Cheese

4 Greek Γαλιον   Latin, Gallium Spanish, Gari Leche blanca Italian French Petit Muguet german, Weiss Walt Dutch

Plate 107

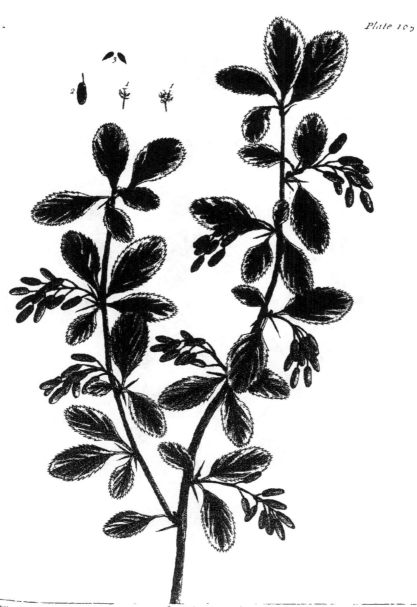

The Barberry Bush.

Eliz Blackwell delin sculp et Pinx

1. Flower
2. Berry open
ed

Berberis vulgaris

Plate 166

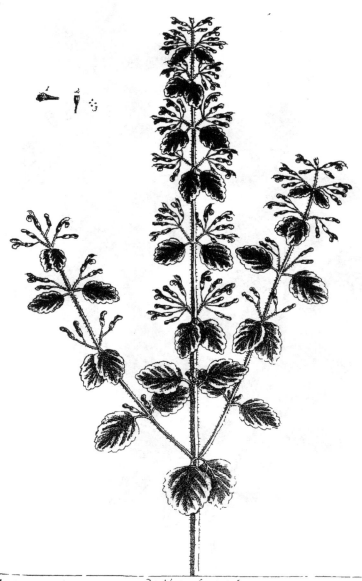

Mountain calamint

Eliz. Blackwell delin. sculp. et n.

1. Flower separate.
2. seed Vessel.
3. seed.

calamintha montana

Plate 229

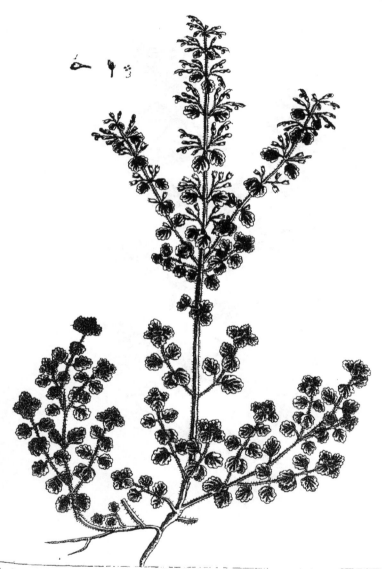

The Common Calamint of the Shops   1 Flower separate   Calamentha officinalis
Eliz Blackwell John sculp et Pinx   2 Seed Vessel open
                                      3 Seed

Plate 168

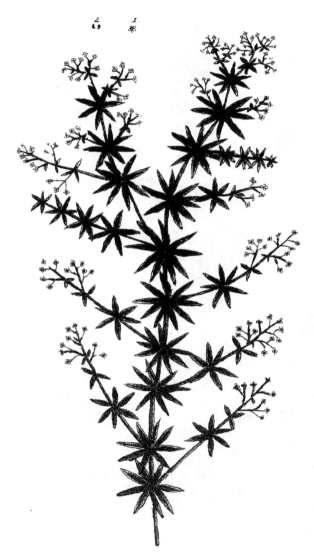

White Ladies Bed Straw

Ebr Blackwell delin. sulp et Pinx

1 Flower
2 Seed

Gallium album latifolium

Mollur illa latifolia.

Plate 169 Golden Rod *Virga aurea*

1. The Stalks grow to be two or three Foot high the Leaves are a light ish green and the Flowers yellow

2. It grows in Woods and Sedges flowering in July

3. The Leaves and Tops are used this being accounted one of our best vulnerary Plants and is much used inwardly in traumatic Apozems and Wound Drinks and outwardly in Cataplasms and Fomentations Some recommend it for spitting of Blood and other Haemorrhages and think it of great Service in the Stone

4. Greek. Latin *Virga aurea angustifolia minus serrata* Spanish Italian *Virga aurea* French *La Vierge doree* german Wundrich Bunder aut Dutch

---

Plate 170 Fluellin or Female Speedwell *Elatine or Veronica femina*

1. This Plant creeps on the Ground with small hairy Stalks about eight Inches long the Leaves are a dark green and the Flowers Purple and yellow

2. It grows in corn Fields and flowers the latter End of Summer

3. This is a vulnerary Plant being accounted good for old Ulcers and spreading cancerous Sores Fluxes Haemorrhages and Inflammations of the Eyes

4. Greek Ἐλατίνη Latin, *Elatine* Spanish, Italian *Elatina* French german Ehrenpreiss Beible Dutch.

Plate 171 Motherwort or Marrubium called *Cardiaca Cardiaca*

1. It grows to be eighteen Inches high, the Leaves are a dark green on the Face and light on the Back, and the Flowers a red Purple

2. It grows in Waste Places and Lanes, flowering in June

3. This Plant, from a supposition that it relieves the Disorders of the heart as a Palpitation and Swooning, takes the Name of Cardiaca Doctor Bowles has commended a Decoction of it sweetned with Sugar as a singular Remedy for the above Illness and for Affections of the Spleen and Hysteric Fits The Powder given in Wine to the Quantity of a Dram is commended as a present Remedy to expediate the Birth

4. Greek, Πράσιον Latin *Marrubium Cardiaca dictum* Spanish Margo Italian Cardiaca French gripaume german Herkgesper Dutch.

Plate 172 Garden Parsly *Apium hortense or Petroselinum vulgare*

1. It grows to be two Foot high, the Leaves are a light grass green and the Flowers white

2. It is sown in gardens and flowers for several Months in y Summer according to the time it is sown

3. The whole Plant is opening attenuating diuretic usefull for Obstructions of the Liver and Spleen, helps the Jaundice, provokes Urine and eases the Stone, gravel and Stranguiry The officinal Preparation is, the Simple Water

4. Greek Σέλινον κηπάιον Latin *Petroselinum vulgare* Spanish Perexel Italian Petrosemolo French Persil de Jardin german Peterlin Dutch

Plate 169

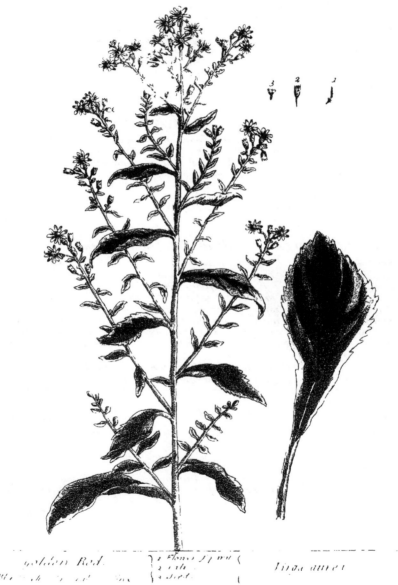

Golden Rod.

Plate 170

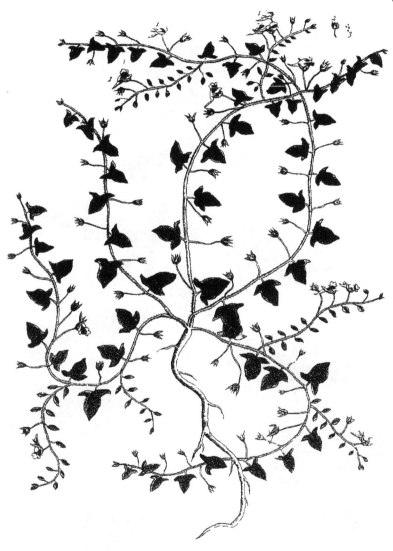

Elatine or Female Speedwell

G. D. Ehret delin. Pinx. & Sculp.

Elatine Female Speedwell

Plate 171

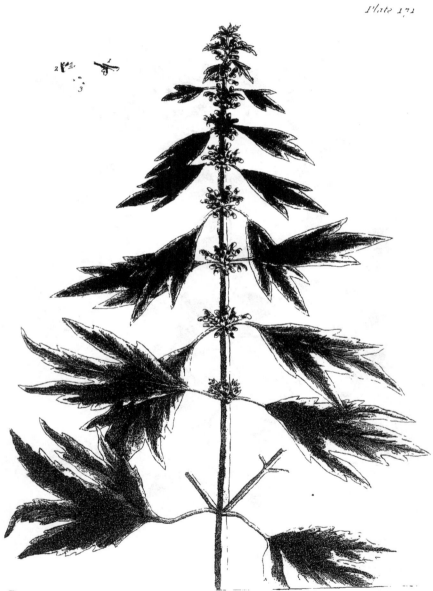

Motherwort. Marrubium alba turi

ruz Bla hn Hl.Chi culp.et Pinx

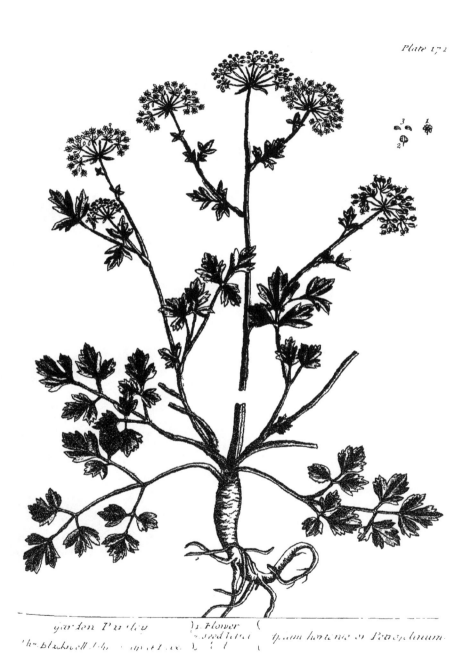

Plate 172

3   1
2

garden Parsley   1. Flower
                      2. seed
The Blackwell del.   3.   Apium hortense or Petroselinum

Plate 173 *The Common Service Tree Sorbus terminalis*

1 This Tree grows pretty tall the Leaves are a light grass Green the Flowers a very pale Yellow and the Berries red

2 It grows in Woods and Thickets, flowring in May but the Fruit is not ripe till October or November

3 The Fruit is accounted restringent and binding good for all kinds of Fluxes either of Blood or Humors, when ripe it promotes Digestion and prevents the too hasty Passage of the Food into the Bowels, some commend it in Fevers attended with a Diarrhed

4 Greek, Oüa Latin, Sorbus vulgaris Spanish, Sorbas   Italian Sorbo salvatico French Sorbes sauvage German Eberaschen Bogelbeer Dutch Wilde Qualster

---

Plate 174 *The Manur'd Service Tree   Sorbus sativa.*

1 This Tree grows much to the same Height as the former, the Leaves are a light the Flowers the same Green on the Face & somewhat hoary on ȳ Back, and the Fruit a redish Brown

2 It grows wild in Staffordshire and Cornwal flowring in May the Fruit being ripe in November

3 The Fruit when green is very restringent, and useful for all kinds of Fluxes This Fruit is seldome to be met with in our Markets, which obliges many to make Use of the former Service Tree in the Place of this

4 Greek, Oüa Latin, Sorbus legittima Spanish, Sorbas Italian Sorba French, Cormes German Sperbern Dutch Tame Qualster

---

Plate 175 *The Bay Tree   Laurus*

1 The Bay Tree seldom grows to any great Bigness here, the Leaves are a dark Green above & a pale underneath ȳ Flowers are yellowish and the Berries Black

2 It grows wild in Spain, Italy and France flowring in May the Fruit being ripe in October

3 The Leaves and Berries are accounted heating, drying and emollient good for Wind in the Stomach and Bowels helping ȳ Collic comforting ȳ Head and Nerves preventing Infections, provoking Urine & the Menses & expelling ȳ Secundines outwardly they are used in Warming and Strengthening Fomentations & Ointments Officinal Preparations are the Elect de Baccis Lauri, Emp de Baccis Lauri and the Oleum Laurinum

4 Greek, Δάφνη Latin Laurus latifolia major Spanish Laurel Italian Lauro French Laurier German Lorberbaum Dutch Laurierboom

---

Plate 176 *Coriander   coriandrum*

1 It grows to be two or three Foot high the Leaves are a bright green and the Flowers white

2 It grows wild in some Places but is commonly sown for the Benefit of the Seed flowring in June

3 The Seed is esteem'd to strengthen the Stomach & expell Wind & is frequently used to correct strong purging Medicines some account it good for the hadns Evil

4 Greek Κόριον η Κοριαννον Latin coriandrum majus vulgare Spanish Culiandro Italian Coriandolo French Coriandre vermicoriandre Dutch Coriander

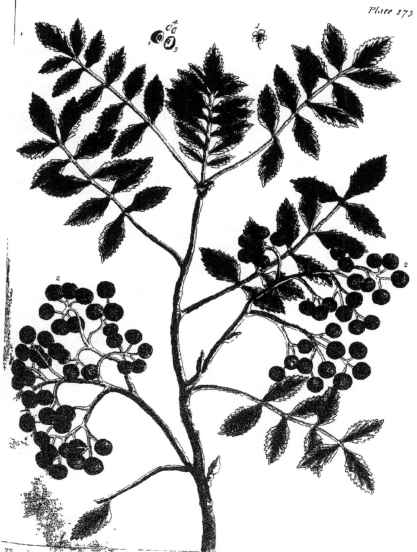

Plate 173

The common Service Tree

Eliz: Blackwell delin: sculp: et pinx:

Plate 174

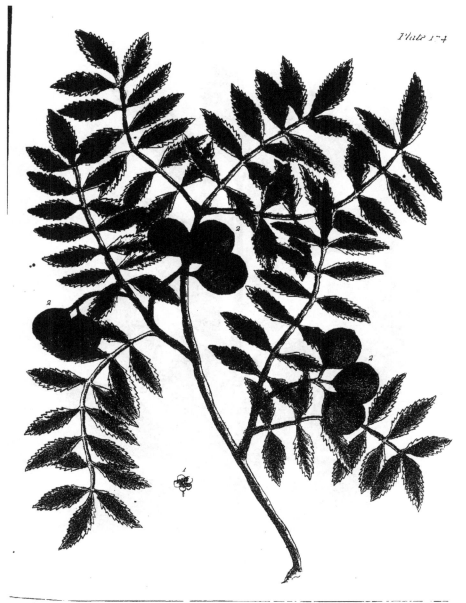

The Manured Service Tree   { 1 Leaves }   Sorbus sativa
Eliz Blackwell delin sculp et Pinx   { 2 Fruit }

Plate 175.

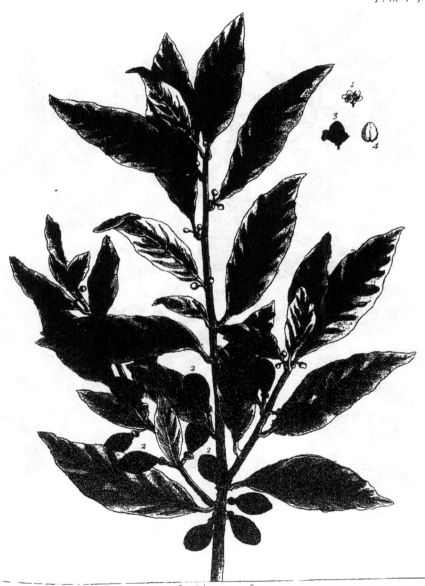

The Bay Tree

1 Flower
2 Fruit
3 Fruit new
4 Kernell

Laurus

E Blackwell delin. Sculp et Pinx.

Plate 176.

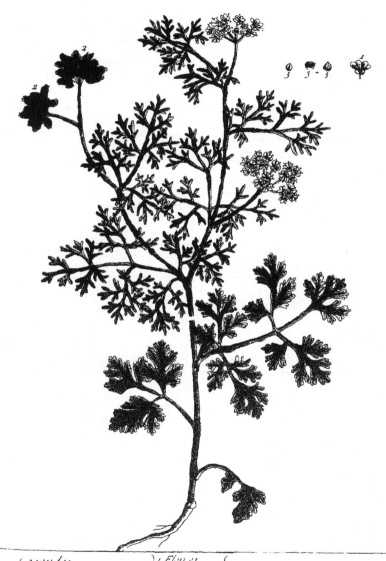

coriander

Nz Blackwell d lin culp i Pinx

1 Flower
2 seed Vessel
3 Seed

coriandrum

Plate 177 Garden Succory Cichorium sativum or Seris
1. It grows to be a Yard high, the Leaves are a grass green and the Flowers blue
2. It is planted in gardens and flowers commonly in June and July
3. Most of the Ancients say that this Plant is cold but its Bitterness shews it to be hot, and is esteem'd aperative, diuretic opening Obstructions of the Liver & helping the Jaundice It also provokes Urine and cleanses of Urinary Parts of slimy Humors The Officinal Preparation is the Syrupus de Cichorio cum Rhabarbaro
4. Greek Σέρις ἀγρία ἥμερος Latin, Seris and Intibus sylvestris Spanish, Almerones Italian, Cichoria domestica French Cichorée German, Begwerse Begwurk Dutch, Cichoren

Plate 178 The Wilding or Crab Tree Malus sylvestris
this tree grows smaller than the garden Apple the Leaves and Blossomes are much the same in colour
It grows in Hedges and flowers in April and May
The use is made of the Juice of the Fruit which is styptic and Binding good for astringent Gargles, Ulcers in the Mouth and Throat and falling down of ye Uvula Outwardly it is good for Burns Scalds Inflammations St Anthonys Fire and red inflammed Eyes
, Greek, Μῆλον ἄγριον Latin, Malus sylvestris Spanish, Maujanas Italian, Mele salvatico French Pomes sauvages German Bild Depffell Dutch, Wilde Appelen

Plate 179 Wall-Flower Leuc. cheir
1. It grows two Foot high, the Leaves are a blue Green and the Flowers yellow
2. It grows upon old Walls and flowers in March and April
3. The Flowers are cordial and cephalic, strengthen the Nerves, help the Apoplexy and Palsy ease the Green-Sickness and procure the Menses The officinal Preparation is the Oil by Infusion of the Flowers which is warming comforting and used for Pains in the Limbs
Greek, Λευκόϊον το φον Latin Leucojum luteum vulgare Spanish Violeta Italian, Viola gialla French, Violets German wilde Regel Beil Dutch

Plate 180 Small Germander Chamaedrys Trifago
1. It grows about eight Inches high, the Leaves are a deep green & the Flowers a red Purple
2. It grows here in gardens and flowers in June and July
3. this Plant is accounted warm, opening Obstructions of the Liver Spleen and Kidneys, helping the Jaundice, Dropsy and Stoppage of Urine Some cry it up as a Specific for the gout Rheumatism and Pain in the Limbs
4. Greek Χαμαίδρυς Latin Chamaedrys minor Spanish Chamedree Italian calamandrina French germandree German gamanderle Dutch Bathenael

No. 45

Plate 177

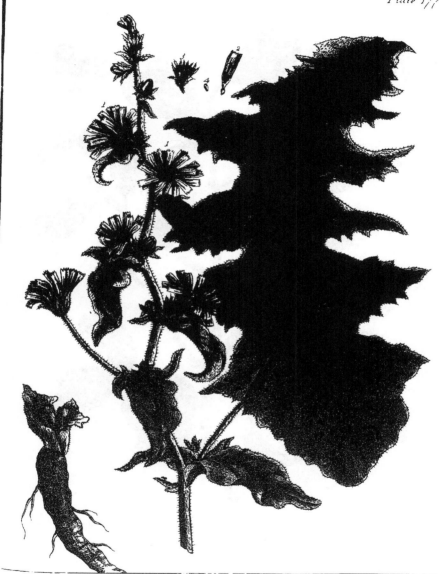

garden Succory

Blackwell del. lin. sculp. et Pinx.

1 Flower
2 Flower separate
3 Calix
4 Seed

Cichorium sativum v Sem

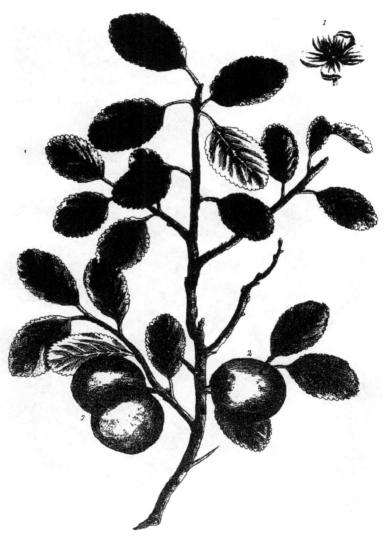

The Wilding wood Tree   1 Blossome   Malus sylvestris
Eliz Blackwell delin sculp et Pinx   2 Fruit.

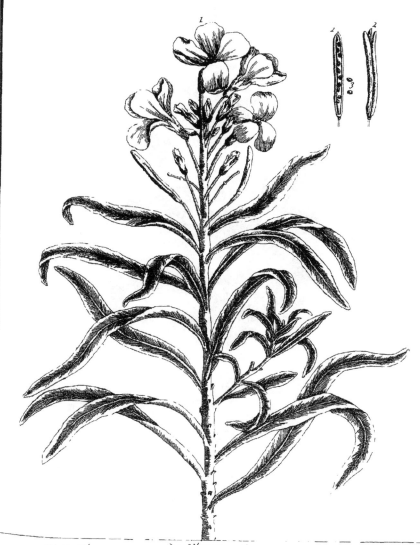

Plate 179

Wall Flower.   1 Flower   Keiri theon
                2 Pod open
Eliz Blackwell delin.   sculp et Pinx   Sciet

Plate 183

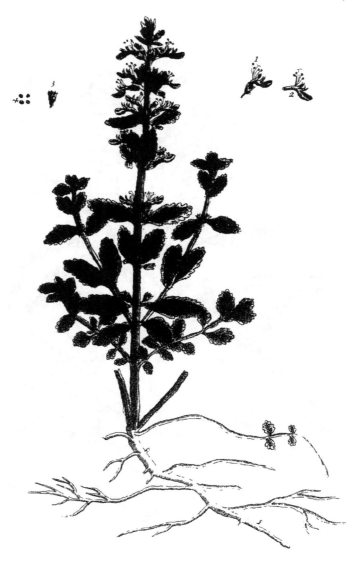

1. Flower
2. Flower opened
3. Cilix
4. Seed

Plate 181 White Stock July flower Leucojum album

1 It grows about two Foot high the Leaves are a light green and the Flowers sometimes White, and often Red and White
2 It is planted in Gardens and flowers most Months in the Summer
3 Dioscorides commends the Flowers for Ulcers & Chaps in ye Fundament & Inflammations of the Matrix Galen says that they help ye Infirmities of ye Liver & Spleen, and provoke the Terms, and hasten the Birth
4 Greek, Λδκοϊον Latin, Leucojum album et purpureum Spanish, Violetas blanguas et amarithas Italian Viola bianca & pavonazza French, Violetz blanches & rouges German Rot Braun und weiss Beil Dutch,

Plate 182 Red Archangel Lamium rubrum

1 This Archangel is much less than the White the Leaves are a grass Green, and the Flowers a pale Purple
2 It grows commonly by Highways and Hedges flowring the greatest part of the Year
3 This Archangel is accounted as great a Specifick for the Excess of ye Catamenia and all Haemorrhages as the White Archangel is for the Fluor Albus Some commend it for great Service in Wounds & Inflammations when outwardly applyed
4 Greek, Γαλιοψις κ Γαλεοβδολον Latin Lamium purpureum, foetidum or Galeopsis purpurea Spanish Ortica muerta bermeja Italian Ortica fetida French, Ortie rouge german Daubnessell Dutch Dove Neetelen

Plate 183 Wild Succory Cichorium sylvestre

1 The Stalks of this dont grow so tall as the Garden but are more stubbed & twisted the Leaves are a fine grass Green, and the Flowers a fine Blue
2 It grows in Lanes and by Hedges flowring in July and August
3 The Vertues of this are much the same as the Garden See Plate 177
4 Greek Κιχόριον άγριον Latin Intubus sylvestris spanish Cichoria de Bosque Italian cichoria salvatica French cichoree sauvage german Bild Begwurk Dutch, Cichorey

Plate 184 Mysseltoe Viscum or Viscus quernus

1 This Plant takes root on the Branches of Trees and sometimes grows two or three Foot long The Leaves are a yellow green the Flowers Yellow and ye Berries almost the colour of white currans
2 It grows upon several Trees as the Apple and Hasel Ash Mapple Lime Willow White thorn & Oak The last of which is hardly to be met with here in England which perhaps added to ye Honour that the Ancient Druids paid this Misseltoe
3 Misseltoe is accounted Cephalic and nervine particularly useful for all kinds of Convulsion Fits, the Apoplexy Palsu and Vertigo, for which Purposes some commend the Misseltoe of the Hasel as better than ye Others The Viscus Aucupum or Bird Lime was formerly made of the Berries of this Plant, but now in England it is made of the Bark of ye Holly Tree Bird Lime is a powerfull Attractive good to ripen hard Tumours and swellings See Sir John Colebatches Discourse of Misseltoe
4 Greek Ιξος Latin Viscum Spanish Viso Italian Vischio or Panio French uuy german, Bogelleim Dutch,

No. 46

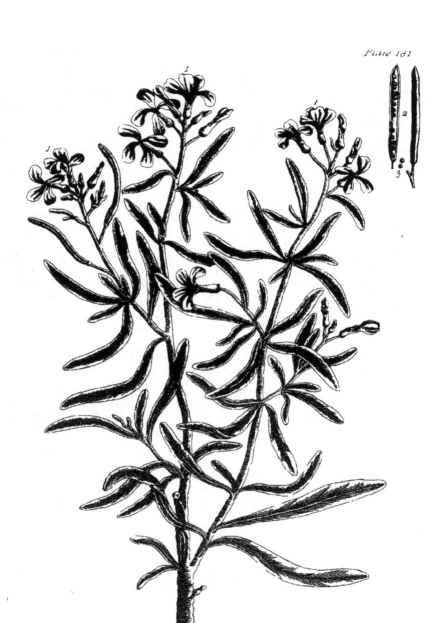

Plate 181

White Stock July flower   1. Flower   Leucoium album
1 2 Blackwell delin sculp et Pinx   2 Pod
     3 Seed

Plate 182

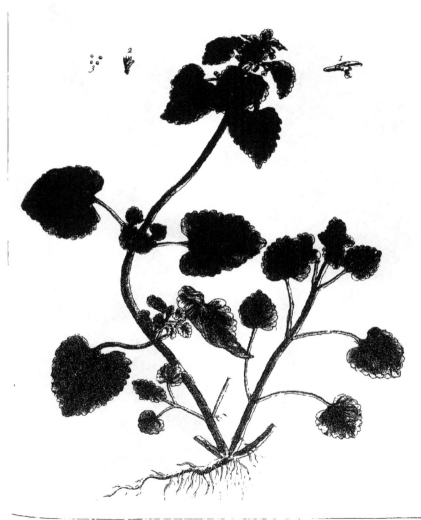

Red Archangel

1 Flower apart
2 Calix
3 Seed

Lamium rubrum

Fhz Blacknell delin sculpt Pinx

Plate 183

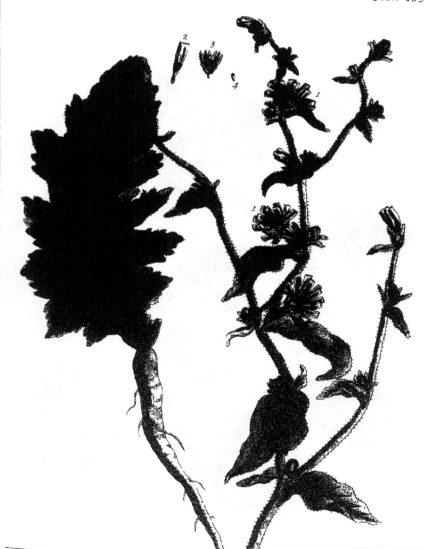

Wild Succory

1 Flower
2 Flower *separate*
3 *calix*
4 *seed*

cichorium sylvestre

Eliz. Blackwell del. sculp et Pinx

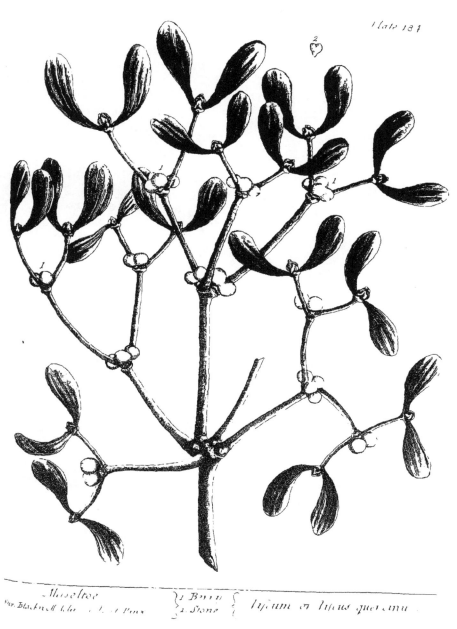

Plate 184

2

1

1

1

Miseltoe

Var. Blackwell del. et sculp. et Pinx. {1 Berry { Viscum or Viscus quercinu
2 Stone

Plate 185 Field Scabious Scabiosa vulgaris pratensis

1 The Stalks grow to be two or three Foot high the Leaves are a grass green and the Flowers purple
2 It grows in Meadows and flowers in June
3 The Leaves are esteem'd cordial alexipharmic sudorific pectoral good for Distempers of the Lungs as Coughs, shortness of Breath &c as also sore Throats and Quinsies Outwardly they are serviceable in the Itch, scabby Sores, Tetters and other cutaneous Distempers They also take black and blue Marks out of the Skin
4 Greek γ Latin Scabiosa Spanish.   Italian Scabiosa
French. Scabieuse German, Apostemen Craut Dutch. Scabiense

Plate 186 The Scarlet Oak Ilex coccigera

This is a small shrubby Oak with prickly Leaves, on the Twigs of which grow little round Grains or rather Nests of Insects of a shining reddish Colour about as big as Peas, made by small Flies These Nests are gathered while they are full of little Worms, and being beat in a Mortar, the Scarlet Liquor is strain'd thro' a Sieve, and mixt with its equal Weight of Sugar which is the Succus Kermes of the Shops
2 It grows in the southern Parts of France Italy and Turky
3 The Succus Kermes is accounted cordial, moderately binding comforting ÿ Heart chearing the Animal Spirits and good to prevent Miscarrying It also drives out the small Pox and Measles
4 Greek. Κόκκος Βαφικη Latin Ilex aculeata cocciglandifera Spanish Grana in Grano Italian. Grana da tingere French. Vermullon German, Scharlachbeer Dutch Scharlaaken Besien Boom

---

Plate 187 The Juniper Tree Juniperus

1 This seldome grows to any great Bigness in England the Leaves are a bluish green, the Flowers a greenish Yellow and the Berries black
2 It grows upon Heaths and flowers in May and June, the Berries are green the first Year and ripe the Second
3 The Wood, Berries and Gum are used the Wood is accounted hot dry and cephalic good to burn in times of Pestilence & contagious Distempers The Berries are esteemed carminative diuretic expelling Wind and usefull in the Stone, gravel & stoppage of Urine the Fume of the Gum is said to be good for Catarrhs. & serous Defluxions up in the Nose and Eyes The Officinal Preparation is the Distill'd Oil
4 Greek. Αρκευθις Latin, Juniperus vulgaris Spanish, Enebro Italian ginepro French, Geneure German, Bectholter Dutch. Deneber Boom

---

Plate 188 The Ivy Tree Hedera arborea

1 This Shrub climbs upon any Thing it grows to the Leaves are a deep green ÿ Flowers yellow and the Berries black
2 It grows in Hedges & flowers in September, ÿ Berries being ripe in January & February
3 The Leaves are accounted good for Inflammations in Issues Scabs Sores & scald Heads Mr Boyle commends a large Dose of the full ripe Berries as a Remedy against ÿ Plague The Gum is said to take spots and Freckles out of the Face
4 Greek Κισσος Latin Hedera Spanish Eda or Hedera Italian Iellera or hedera French Lierre german Ranes Dutch klimop Boombyl

No 47

Plate 105.

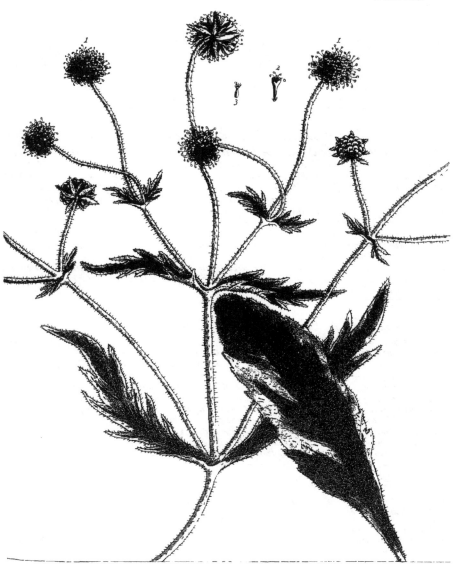

Wild *Sialdours*

Fhx Blacknell delin sulp.e Pins

{ 1 Flower
2 Flower apart }
{ 3 seed

Scabious sylvestris

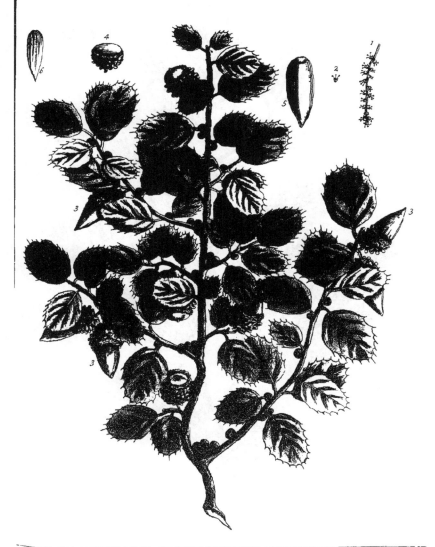

Plate 186

The Scarlet Oak

Blackwell when . . .

1 catkin 2 flower, . . .
3 fruit 4 cup
5 kernel of fruit

Plate 107

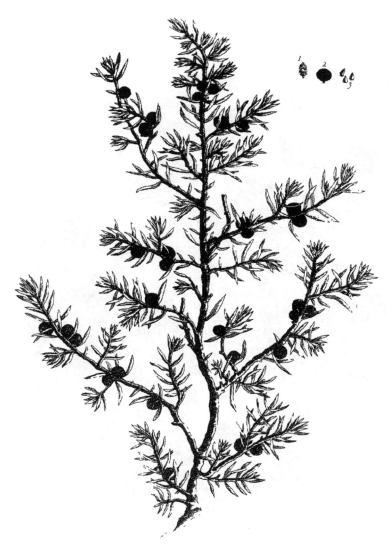

The Juniper Tree   Genévrier
the Fl...   1 Bou...   Juniperus

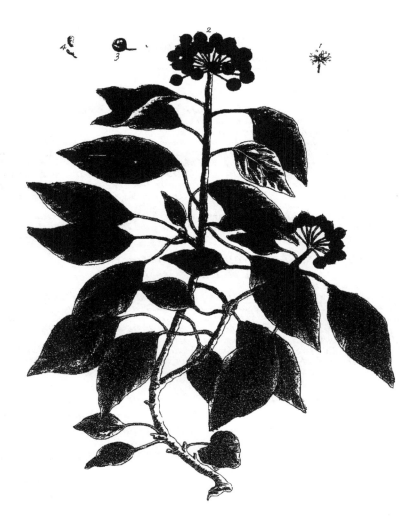

The Ivy Tree   *1 Flower*   *Hedera arborea*
The Black Ivie with cup or Cæce   *2 Berries*

Plate 189 *The Pine Tree or manur'd Pine Pinus or Pinus sativa*

1 This is a large Tree with slender sharp pointed dark green Leaves yellow catkins and brown oblong round pointed Cones

2 It grows wild in Italy but is planted here in gardens flowering early in the Spring

3 The Nucles or Kernels are of a balsamic nourishing Nature and esteem'd good for consumptions coughs and Hoarsness restorative and of Service after long Illness They also help ye Stranguary Heat & Sharpness of Urine

4 Greek Πιτυς Latin Pinus Spanish Pino Italian Pino French Pin german Fichtenbaum Dutch Pyn Boom

----

Plate 190 *The wild Pine Pinus sylvestris*

1 This Pine grows near as tall as the former, its Leaves are much shorter and slenderer especially on the Bottom of the Branches, the catkins & Cones smaller and sharper, but much of the same colour

2 It grows in great Plenty in Germany & flowers much about ye time with the other

3 From this Tree comes the common Turpentine chiefly used by the Farriers, from which is distill'd the oil of Turpentine and the Spirit, the Dregs that are left at the Bottom of the Still is the common Rosin Mr Dale affirms from Doctor Kreig that ye Burgundy Pitch is made of ye Turpentine from this Tree The curious may Consult Mr Miller the Apothecary's Botanicum officinale p 347 where there is a lengthfull Account of this Tree

4 greek Πιτυς αγρια Latin Pinus montana Spanish Pino de bosque Italian Pino pilvatico French Pin sauvage german Bildfichtenbaum Dutch Wilde Pynboom

----

Plate 191 *Orpine or Live-long Crassula or Fabaria*

1 The Stalks grow to be a Foot high, the Leaves are a light blue green and the Flowers a pale Purple

2 It grows in Hedges and shady Places flowering in June and July

3 The Leaves and Flowers are accounted cooling and binding good for the bloody Flux tempering the Heat and Acrimony of those Humours which cause an Erosion of the Bowels Outwardly they are used against Burns and Scalds, and all kinds of Inflammations

4 Greek Τελεφιον Latin Telephium vulgare Spanish   Italian Fava maior French Reprise or Joubarbe des Vignes german Schmeerwurkel Dutch Smeernote

----

Plate 192 *Featherfew Matricaria*

1 The Stalks grow about two Foot high the Leaves are a yellow green the Flowers white with a yellow Thrum in the Middle

2 It grows in Hedges and Lanes flowering in June and July

3 This Plant is particularly appropriated to the Female Sex being of great Service in all cold flatulent Disorders of the Womb and hysteric Affections provoking the catamenia and expelling the Birth and Secundines about two Ounces of the Juice taken an Hour before the Fit is good in all kinds of Agues It also destroys Worms provokes Urine and helps in Dropsy and Jaundice

4 Greek Παρθενιον Latin Parthenium Spanish   Italian Maria or Amarella French Matricaire german Reinfart Dutch Moderkruid

Plate 103

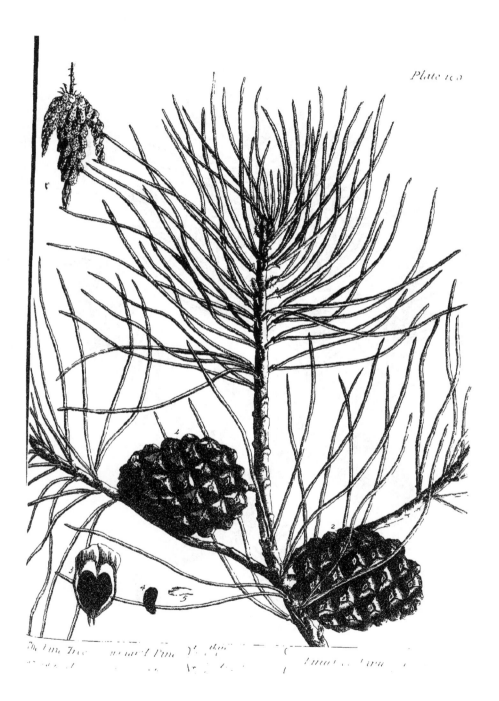

The Pine Tree   Scrub Pine

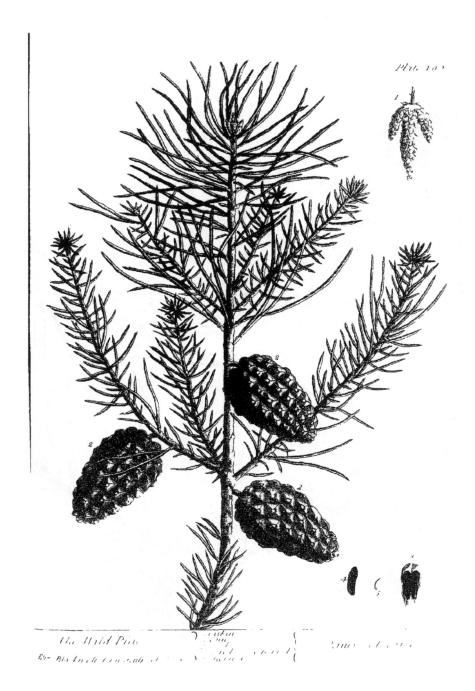

Plate 10

The Wild Pine

E— Black heath branch . . . .

Plate 101

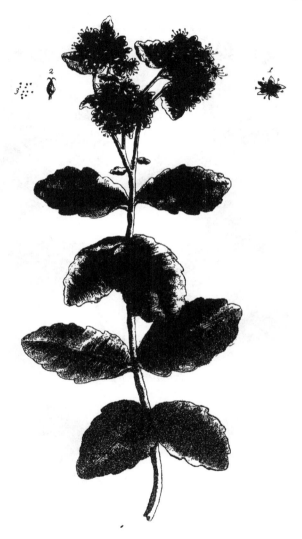

Orpine or Live long
Ilz Blz knell delar culp et Puix
1 Flower
2 Seed Vessel
3 Seed

Plate 162

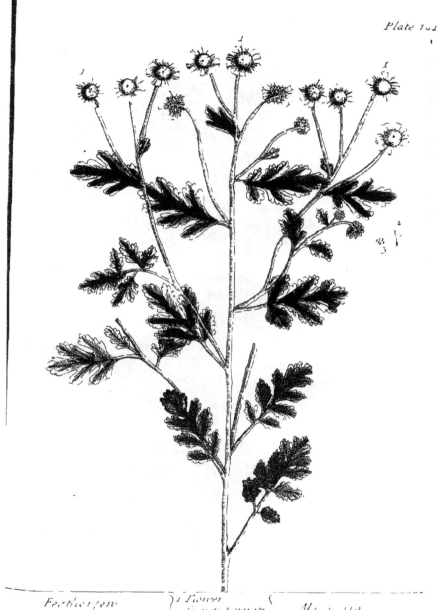

Feverfew   ) 1 Flower   (
) Flower lemarate   (Motherwort
     2 Blet   s e n cal s mm)   (

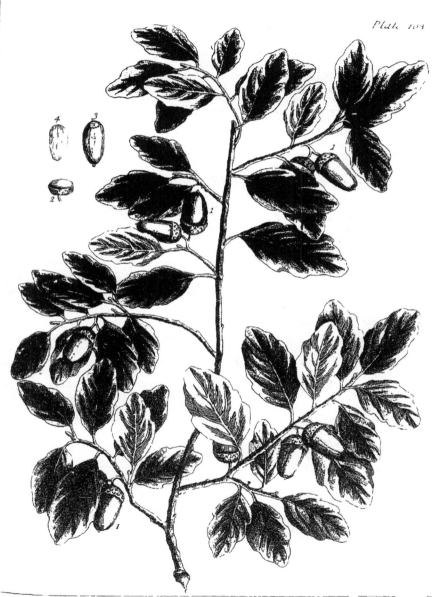

Plate 108

The Cork Tree

Plate 193 The Cork Tree Suber

1. This is a kind of ever green Oak its Leaves are thicker and much less indented than the common Oak, and the Acorns smaller
2. It grows in Spain and Italy and the Southern Parts of France
3. The Bark of which they make Cork is separated from the Tree by making a long Incision from the Head to the Root of the Tree which they take care to do in dry Weather, for the young tender Bark is lyable to be destroyed and the Trees killd by Rain Cork is said to be restringent and good for all kinds of Fluxes some commend the Ashes or burnt Cork, for the same Purposes
4. Greek Φελλὸς Latin Suber latifolium perpetuo virens Spanish Italian Sugaro French German Pantoffelholtz Dutch Kurck

Plate 194 The Bay of Alexandria Laurus Alexandrina

1. The Stalks are tough & limber seldom growing to any great height the Leaves are a light Green the Flowers are greenish with a purple Umbo in the Middle
2. It grows in the Mountainous Parts of Italy and in Hungary
3. Dioscorides and Galen recommend it to open Obstructions of the kidneys & the Womb to provoke Urine & the Menses, and to help long & hard Labour some account it a good vulnerary Plant, & useful to dry up old Ulcers and Sores
4. Greek Δάφνη Ἀλεξανδρεία Latin Laurus Alexandrina genuina Spanish Italian Lauro Alysandrino French Laurier Alexandrin German Dutch

Plate 195 The Mastich or Lentisk-Tree Lentiscus

1. This Tree grows to a considerable Bigness in its native Soil the Leaves are a dark grass green the Flowers a greenish Yellow and the Berries black
2. It grows in the Southern Parts of France and in Italy but it yields the gum Mastich only in the Island of Scio, or Chio in the Archipelago
3. The Gum is esteem'd heating & drying strengthning the Head & Nervous System & Stomach it eases a tough tops spitting of Blood & stays Vomiting The Ladies in Turky chew it to preserve the gums & Teeth & procure a Sweet Breath Gum and by it is used in Plaisters for the Head Ach & Tooth-Ach The Wood is accounted drying & binding good for all kinds of Fluxes
4. Greek Σχῖνος Latin Lentiscus vulgaris Spanish Mata o' Irvina Italian Lentasco French Lentisque German Mastixbaum Dutch Mastix Boom

Plate 196 The Box Tree Buxus

1. Box seldom grows to any great Bigness here the Leaves are a deep shining green the Flowers yellow and the Fruit a browinish green
2. It grows wild in some Parts of Kent & Surry at Box hill near Dorking
3. Some commend the chips of the Wood, or the Tree Tenerea in .... in ... leaves and is of the same Nature The Oil distilled from the Wood ... ... of the Tooth-Ach a little Lint or cotton being dipt in it & put into a hollow tooth
4. Greek Πύξος Latin Buxus arborescens Spanish Italian bosso French Buis German Dutch Palmboom

Plate 193

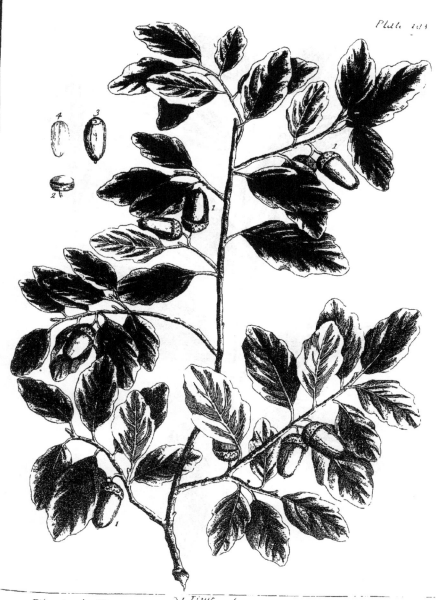

The Cork Tree

Plate 154

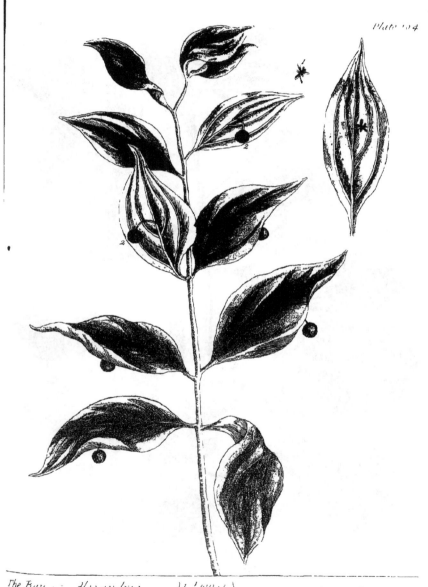

The Bay of Alexandria

Blackwell del. sculp. et Pinx.   Laurus Alexandrina

Plate 10

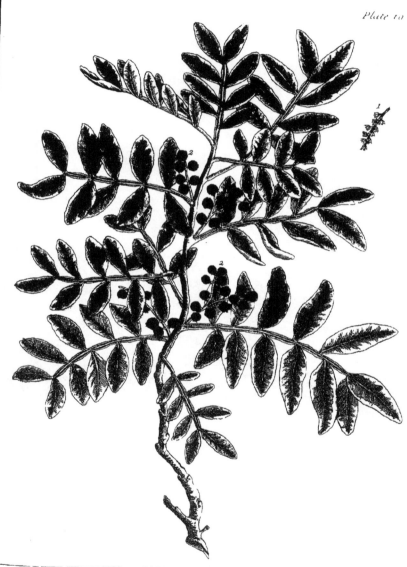

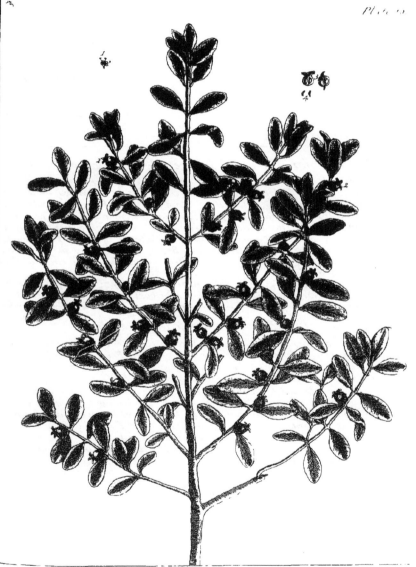

The Box Tree

Ther Blackn. delin. sculp.

197 The true sweet gum cistus of Candy Cistus ladanifera vera cretica

This Shrub grows to be two or three Foot high the Leaves are a grass Green the Flowers a pale Red with a large purple spot in ÿ End next the Seed Vessel

It grows in ÿ Island of Candy & other places in ÿ Archipelago & flowers in Iuly

From this Tree comes the Gum Labdanum of ÿ Shops which some commend as good for a Looseness & Gripes caused by sharp Humours The Fume of it comforts the Brain, & stops catarrhous Defluxions Outwardly applied it is accounted strengthening to the Stomach and stays Vomiting See Mr Ioseph Miller Botanicum Officinale p 252 & 253

Greek Κισ☉ ν Κιδαϑον, ἡ Κιαραϑον Latin Cistus Ledan Cetense Spanish Ierguados Italian, Cisto French, German.
Dutch Labdanum Boom

Plate 198 The Common Fir or Pitch Tree Abies rubra or Picea

This grows to be a large Tree, the Leaves are small slender & prickly, of a bright grass Green colour the Catkins greenish, the Cones a light Brown & ÿ Seed Brown

It grows wild in Germany & Scotland sending out its Catkins in the Spring

The Leaves and Tops are used in Diet Drinks for the Scurvy & are an Ingredient in the Brunswick Mum The Strasburg Turpentine comes from this Tree, which is mollifying healing & cleansing & a great Diuretic usefull in Wounds Ulcers a gonorrhea the Fluor albus, the Stone & Gravel & Affections of ÿ Breast & Lungs Tar is also the Product of this Tree, and is accounted a good pectoral Medicine, useful for shortness of Breath and Obstructions of the Lungs

Greek Πεύκη Latin Picea Spanish, Pino negro Italian Pezzo French, Pesse Pignet or Garipolt German, Rat Zannenbaum Dutch, Denne Boom

---

Plate 199 The Olive Tree Olea or Olea sativa

This Tree grows to a great Bigness in its native Climate, the Leaves are a deep Green above & hoary underneath, the Flowers yellow & the Fruit black when ripe

It grows in Spain, Italy and Turky

The Oil is moderately healing & mollifying rendering the Body lax & soluble it helps Disorders of ÿ Breast & Lungs & eases Gripings & the Colic It is of great use against all corrosive mineral Poisons as Arsenic Sublimate &c It opens ÿ Urinary Passages & is good for ÿ Stone & Gravel The pickled Olives are grateful to ÿ Stomach and provoke an Appetite The ripe Olives are a great Part of ÿ Food of the Eastern Countries among the Greeks especially in Lent

Greek Ελάια Latin Olea Spanish Olivo or Azeutimo Italian Olivo French Olivier German Dellaum Dutch Oliuf

---

Plate 200 The Small wild Daisy Bellis sylvestris minor

The Stalks grow about four Inches high, the Leaves are a light green, the Flowers white set about a yellow Thrum & sometimes red round ÿ Edge & red underneath

It grows in Fields & Meadows flowering in March April and May

This is accounted a traumatic & Vulnerary Plant being used in Wound Drinks the Leaves are esteemed good to dissolve congealed & coagulated Blood help ÿ Pleurisy and Peripneumony Some commend a Decoction given Inwardly and a Cataplasm of ÿ Leaves applied outwardly as extraordinary Remedies in the Hip Evil

Greek   Latin Bellis minor Spanish   Italian Fior de
vera French Pasquette Pasquier German Madelen Dutch Maatliefen
p. 50

Plate 197

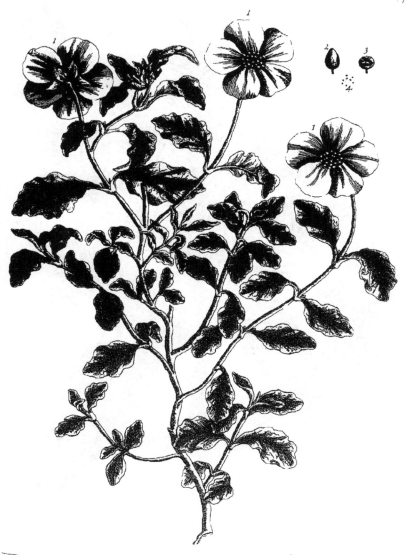

1. Sweet Althea of Candia
2. Bladen Hannah et Pat

1. Florts
2. Seed Vessel and the seeds
3. Seed
4. Seed

Plate 198

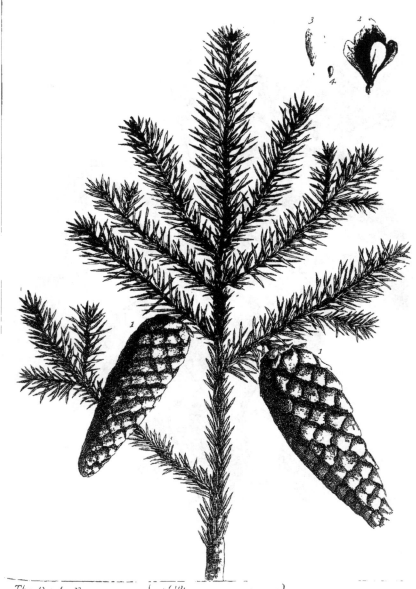

The Pitch Tree

the Black Adder cully above

Pi..

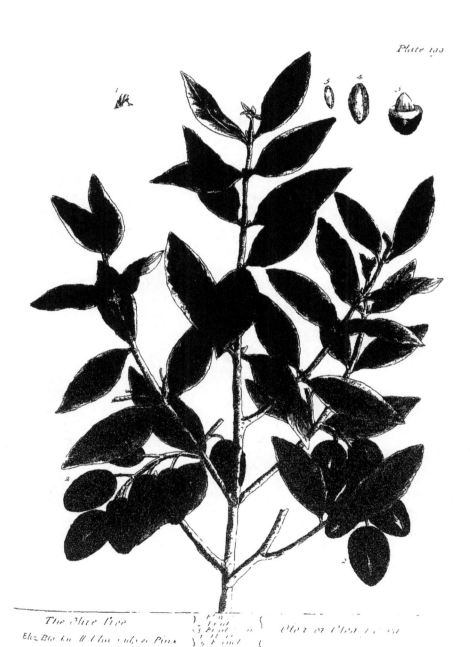

Plate 190

The Olive Tree

Elæ Blo ku W blw cul, ei Pin.x   Oleo or Olea l. 341

Plate 200

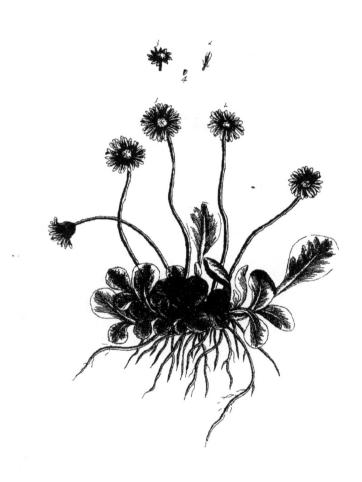

The Small wild Daisy

Bellis sylvestris minor

Plate 201 The Tamarind Tree Tamarindus

1 This is the west India Tamarind the Specimen of the Tree is taken from one in the Stove in y Physick Garden, and the Fruit is taken from the Life out of Mr Rand's Collection This Tree grows very large in the West Indies the Leaves are a light grass Green, the Flowers white & yellow with purple Veins, the Pods a brownish yellow tinctured with Red the Pulp of the Pods is yellow at first & then changes into a brownish black, & the Stones are a reddish shining Brown.

2 It grows in the West Indies, and flowers in Summer

3 These Tamarinds are generally eat by themselves, without any other Medicine mixt with them, and are accounted good to purge choleric Humours, & correct the bilious Heat in the Stomach and Bowels

4 Greek, Οξυφοίνικες Latin, Tamarindus Spanish,   Italian.
French,   German,   Dutch, Tamarinde

Plate 202 The Palm, or Date Tree. Dactilus or Palma

1 This is a large Tree with a rough scaly Bark on the main Stem, the Leaves grow on the Top of the Tree in form of the sticks of a Fan, the Flowers are white, and the Fruit yellow and red

2 It grows in Barbary, Egypt and Syria

3 The Dates are much used for Food in the Countries where they grow here they are esteemd drying and binding, usefull for Fluxes, and to smooth the Roughness of the Aspera Arteria.

4 Greek, Φοίνιξ Latin, Palma. Spanish Palmera Italian Palma French, Palmier German, Dattelbaum Dutch Dadel

---

Plate 203 The male Fir or Silver Fir Abies mas

1 This grows to be very large, the Leaves are broad at the Ends & white underneath and the Cones grow erect

2 This Tree is said to grow wild in some Parts of England, but is found in great Plenty in the mountainous Parts of Germany

3 This is the Tree which ought to be used in the Shops according to the Dispensatory but not being so common as the Spruce, that generally supplies its Place, the Vertues of both being much the same See the Explanation of Plate 108.

4 Greek Ελάτη Latin Abies mas, Conus sui cum spectantibus Spanish, Abeto Italian Abiet German, Dannenbaum Dutch, Denne Boom

---

Plate 204 Colts-foot or Foles-foot Tussilago or Farfara

1 The Stalks on which the Flowers grow are about four Inches high the Leaves are a yellow green above & whitish underneath and the Flowers yellow

2 It grows in moist watery Places and flowers in February & March

3 The Leaves & Flowers are accounted pectoral, good for Diseases of the Lungs and Breast as Coughs Consumptions & shortness of Breath some smoak the dried Leaves among Tobacco for Coughs & Affections of the Lungs

4 Greek Βηχιον Latin, Ungula caballina Spanish, Unha da Asno Italian Farfarella French Pas de Asne German Brantlattich Dutch Hoefbladen

51

Plate 201

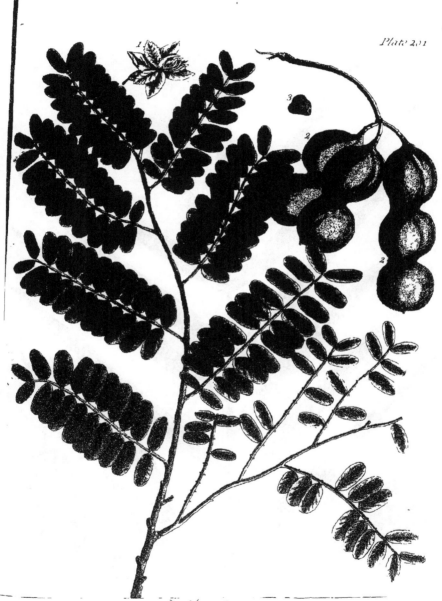

The Tamarind Tree   1 Flower   *Tamarindus*
Flz Brickwell delin culp ad viv   Pod   Stone

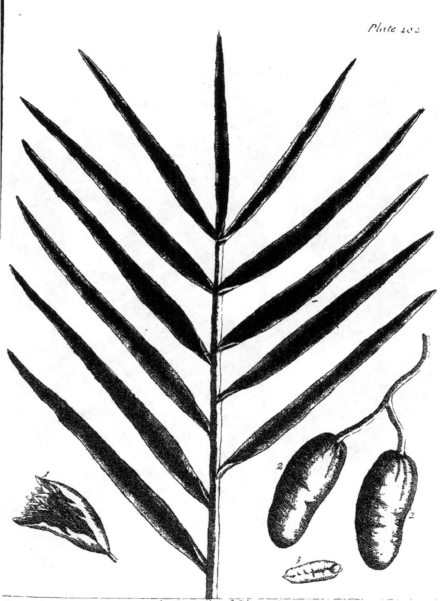

Plate 202

The Palm or Date Tree

1 Fresh or old Flower
2 Fruit
Eliz Blackwell delin sculpet Pinx 3 Stone

Dactylus or Palma

Plate 203

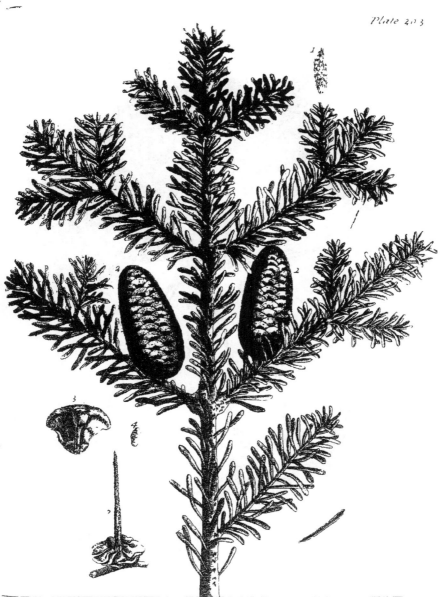

The male Fir or Silver Fir

E. Blackwell delin. sculp. et Pinx.

{
1 catkin
2 Cone
3 a ripe Scale
4 Seed
5 the pith of the cone
}

Abies mas

Plate 2.4

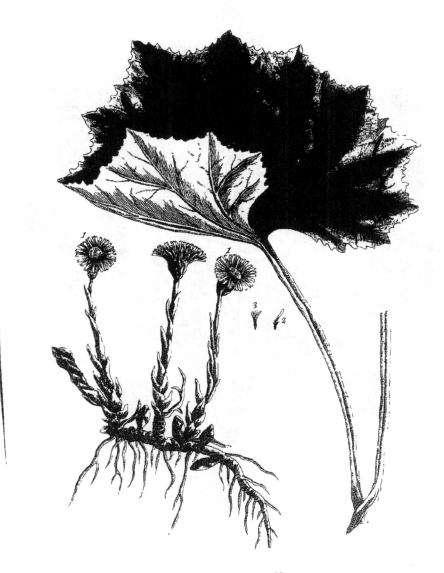

Coltsfoot or Foleusoot } 1 *Flower*
2 *Flower separate* } *Tussilago or Farfara*
Ehz Bla [...] et dPaux } 2 *Seed*

Plate 205. The Holly-Tree Aquifolium

1. This Tree grows to be pretty large, the Leaves are a deep Green the Flowers yellowish, and the Berries red
2. It grows wild in the Warm Countries, and flowers in the Spring
3. From this Tree is made our Bird-lime which is a powerfull attractive & good to ripen hard Tumours & Swellings, & is an Ingredient in Emplastrum Diachilon magnum
4. Greek, Latin, Aquifolium Spanish, Italian Agrifolio French, Houx German, Balddisteln oder Stechpalmen Dutch, Hulst

---

Plate 206 The Magellanic Bay-like Tree or Winter's Bark Cortex Winteranus

1. The Bark of this Tree which is ye Part chiefly used is a brownish Ash colour the Leaves a blue Green, & the Flowers purple succeeded by Green Berries
2. It grows on the Magellanic Coasts
3. This Bark is rarely to be met with in the Shops, it is accounted a specific against the Scurvy, and a good Nervine Medicine, helpfull in Palsies and Convulsions, some account it good for Diseases of the Stomach and Bowels
4. Greek, Latin, Cortex Winteranus, Laurifolia Magellanica Cortice aeri Spanish Italian, French German Dutch,

---

Plate 207 Noble Liverwort Hepatica nobilis.

1. The Stalks grow about four or five Inches high, the Leaves are a grass Green, the Flowers sometimes white, sometimes blue & sometimes a red Purple
2. It is planted in Gardens and flowers in March
3. The Leaves are commended by some foreign Authors as a good Vulnerary and useful in Distempers of the Liver
4. Greek, Latin, Trifolium aureum Spanish, Italian, Herba Trinita French German, Gulden Leberkraut Dutch, Edel Leverkruyd

---

Plate 208 Venetian Orobus The True Orobus Orobus Venetus & Orobus

1. The Plant mark'd with the Figure 1 is the Broad-leaved or Venetian Orobus and has generally a purple Flower. That mark d 2 is the Ervum or bitter Vetch, which is commonly used in the Shops the separate Figures below to this last, for the Seed Pod and Flower of the other are very different, the Seed of the first being black the Pod pretty large & the Flower pale Purple, the Seed of ye other is white the Flower white & the Pod small
2. They grow in Italy and some Parts of France flowring in Iune
3. The Powder of Orobus mixt with Honey is said to cleanse the Lungs of Tough Phlegm and is a strong Diuretic expelling the Stone & gravel, but if tak n too frequently it causes bloody Urine
4. Greek, Opoβos Latin, Ervum & Orobus Alpinus latifolius Spanish, Italian Ervo or Mocho French German Dutch.

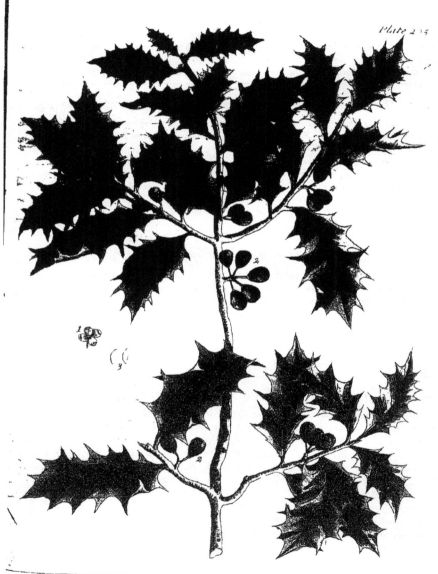

Plate 2 5

The Holly-Tree } 1 Flower { Aquifolium
Fkz Blackwell delin n sp et Pinx } 2 Berry {
} 3 Seed {

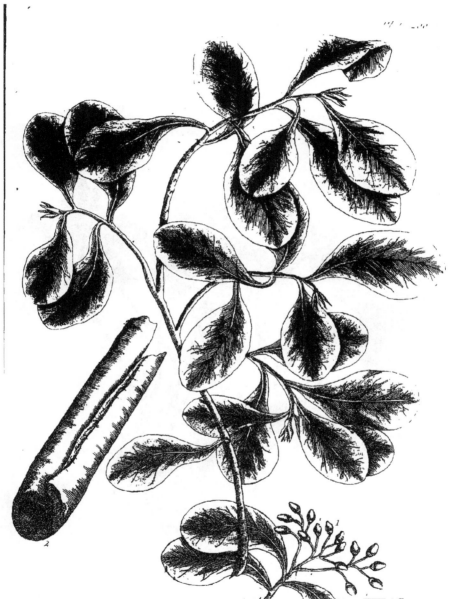

the Magellanic Bay like Tree } 1 *Berries* {
or Winters Bark } 2 *the Bark huell* {

E͞. Blah of the . *de Prin*

Plate 287

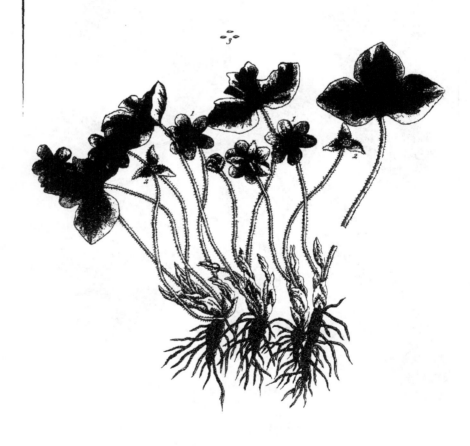

Noble Liverwort

1. Flower
2. Red Vessel
3. Seed

Hepatica nobilis

Eliz Blackwell delin. sculp. et Pinx.

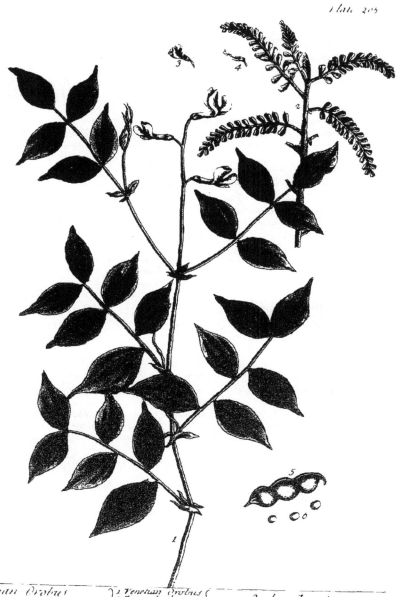

Plate 285

Venetian Orobus
The true Orobus

Eliz. Blackwell del. Sculp. et Pinx.

1 Venetian Orobus
2 True Orobus
3 Flower 4 cut
5 Pod 6 seed

Orobus Tenetus
& Orobus

Plate 209 The Carob Tree Carobe or Siliqua

This Tree grows to a considerable Bigness in its native Climate the Leaves
are a bright grass Green, the Flowers red the Pods a brownish red, and
the Fruit a deep red

- It grows in Syria & Greet, & flowers in y Spring the Fruit being ripe in Autumn
  Matthiolus recommends the Fruit as good for the Stomach and Griping of y
  guts, & to provoke Urine The Decoction of the Beans is accounted by him a
  great Cure for an inveterate Cough, and the Tissuk
4 Greek, Keράτια Latin, Siliqua Spanish, Alfarbas or Carrouges Italian, Carobole
  French, Carronge German, St Johannis Brode Dutch, Sint Jans Blom

---

Plate 210 The Tree of Life Arbor Vitae

1 It seldome grows to any great Bigness in England, the Leaves resemble
  much those of y Cypress Tree, & the Cones are a light Brown
2 Its native Climate is Canada
3 The Leaves are accounted digesting and attenuating Parkinson says they
  have done great Service in freeing the Lungs from thick Flegm, by chewing
  them fasting in the Morning.
4 Greek, Kέδεος λνκια Latin Lycia Cedrus Spanish,   Italian,
  Cedro Lycio French,   German,   Dutch,

Plate 211 Thyme Thymus

1 It grows about half a Foot high, the Leaves are a dark green and the
  Flowers a pale Purple
- It grows wild in Spain and flowers here in July
3 Thyme is esteem'd heating and attenuating good to free the Lungs from viscid
  Flegm and help Wheesing and shortness of Breath It is also accounted
  cephalic and good in all Diseases of the Head & Nerves The Officinal Prepara
  tion is The Oleum Thymi distillatum
4 Greek Θύμος Latin, Thymum durius Spanish, Tomilho salfero. Italian
  Timo French, Tim German, Romischer Duendel Dutch, Thym

Plate 212 Rue leaved Whitlow Grass Paronychia rutaceo folio

1 This Plant seldome exceeds four or five Inches in height the Leaves are
  reddish Green and the Flowers white
2 It grows on the Tops of Walls & flowers in March and April
3 Mr Boyle commends this Plant as a Specific for the Lungs Evil
  St John Colebatch in his Essay upon Acids & Alkalys makes mention of a
  poor Gul in Worcestershire afflicted with Scrophulous Ulcers who received a
  Benefit from it
4 Greek Παρωνυχια Latin Ruta muraria Spanish,   Italian
  Paronichia French,   German, Nanerrauten Dutch,

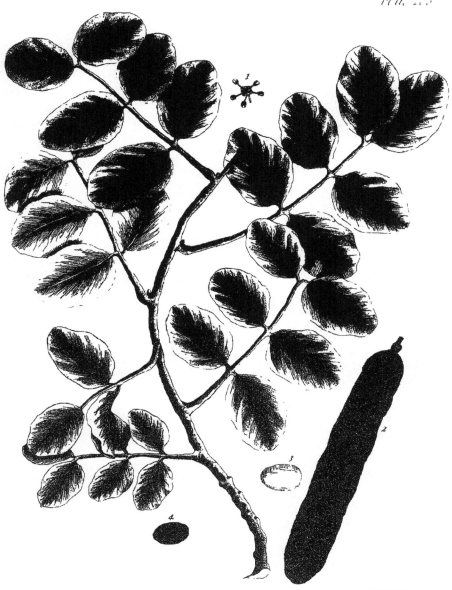

Plate 289

1

2

3

4

The Carob Tree   { 1 Flower   }   Caroba or Siliqua.
                 { 2 Pod   }
Eliz Blackwell delin: sculp: et Pinx { 3 Fruit   }
                         { 4 Stone   }

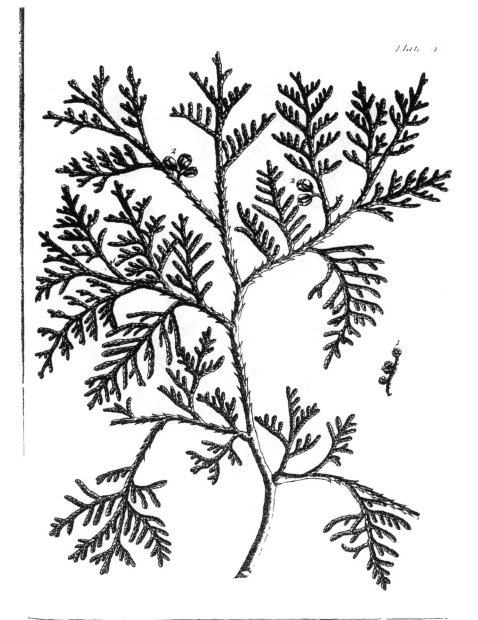

The Tree of Life   { 1 cochin. }   Arbor Vitæ
{ 2 cono }

Ehz Blackwell delin culp et Pinx

Plate 211

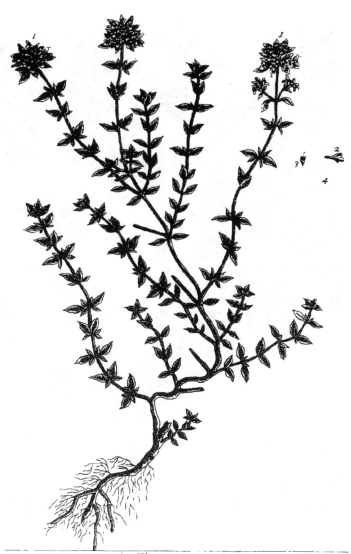

Thyme

Eliz. Blackwell delin. sculp. et Pinx.

1 Flower
2 Flower separate
3 Calex
4 Seed

Thymus

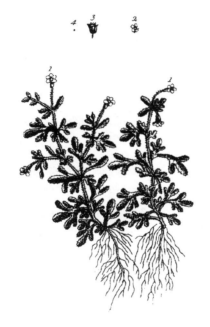

Plate 212

4 3 2

2 1

Rue-leaved Whitlow-Grass

az ceste Whitlow-grass Pins

1 Flower
2 Flower opened
3 calix
4 Seed

Paronichia rutacei folia

Plate 213 *The Wild Olive Tree Olea Sylvestris, or Oleaster*

This Tree grows less than the manur'd Olive the Leaves are narrower than
the Flowers white with a blush of purple in them, & the Fruit black when ripe
It grows in great Plenty in Tuscany and flowers in April
Matthiolus recommends the Leaves & the Wood as binding & cooling Dioscorides saith
the Oil is exceeding astringent, and accounts the Leaves and Fruit good for St
Anthonys Fire and corroding Sores
Greek, Αγριελαια Latin Oleaster Spanish, Zebuche Italian, Olivo salvatico
French, Olivier sauvage German Bilder ollbaum Dutch, Wilde Olyf

Plate 214 *The Savine Tree Sabina*

It seldome grows tall in England the Leaves are a grass Green the Flowers
Green and the Berries a blackish purple
It is planted here in Gardens and seldome produces Fruit for which some
have thought it barren
Savine is accounted hot & dry opening & attenuating being a great Provoker of
the Catamenia causing Abortion & expelling the Birth It is esteemd good to destroy
Worms in Children, for which Purpose Mr Ray commends the Juice mixt with
Milk & sweetned with Sugar the Juice beat into a cataplasm with Hogs Lard,
cures Childrens Scabby Heads Officinal Preparations are the Ul Sabinae per
Infusionem et decoctionem & the Oleum Sab chymicum
Greek, Βραθυς Latin Sabina Spanish Sabina Italian, Savina French,
Savinier German Sebenbaum Dutch Sevenboom

Plate 215 *Wall fern or Polypody of the Oak Polypodium Quercinum*

This Plant grows about eight or ten Inches high on the back of the Leaves grow
the Flowers of a reddish brown colour
It grows on old Walls and Trees and flowers in Autumn
The Roots are esteemd opening & good to purge bilious Humours & open Obstructi-
ons of the Liver, help the Jaundice & Dropsy & provoke Urine. Some account them good in
the Scurvy for which they are frequently an Ingredient in Antiscorbutic Diet Drinks
Greek Πολυποδιον Latin, Filicula Spanish, Polipopio Italian, Polipodio
French, Polypode German, Dropffwurk Dutch, Boomvaren

Plate 216 *Spleen Wort, Ceterach, Miltwast Asplenium, Ceterach, Scolopendrium*

It grows about four Inches high the Leaves are a dark Green on the upper Side &
brownish on the back Side which is occasioned by the Seeds growing there
It grows on old Walls and Buildings
This is one of the five capillary Plants taking its Name from the good Effects which in
curing the Diseases of the Spleen taking away the Swellings, and hindering its too
great Largness whence it is called Miltwast it also opens Obstructions of the Liver
and helps the Jaundice and is good to cure the Rickets in children
Greek Ασπληνιον Latin Asplenium Spanish Doradilha Italian Asplenio & Ceterach
Ceterach German.   Dutch Scolopendria

No 54

Plate 213

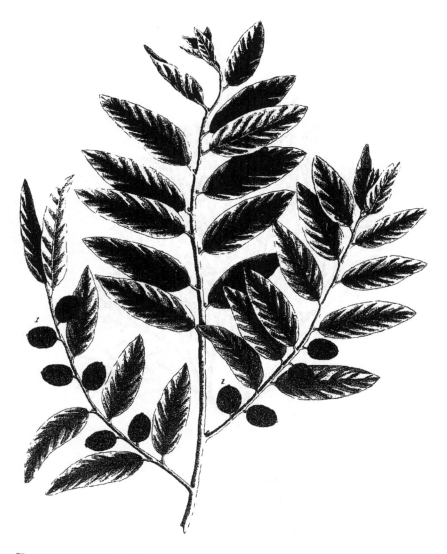

The Wild Olive Tree

Eliz. Blackwell delin sculp et Pinx.

1 Fruit

Olea sylve tris or Eleva ts

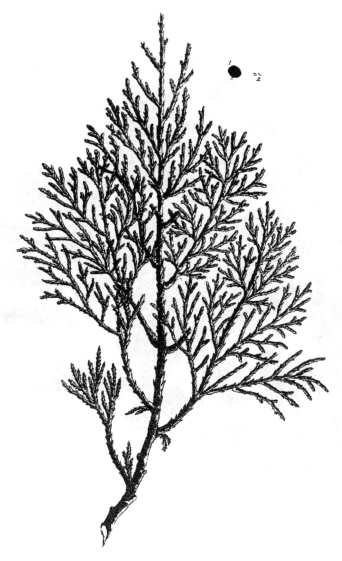

The Savine Tree.
Hæc Bac....tha ...Pini.   } 1 Fruit {   Sabina
                        } Seed {

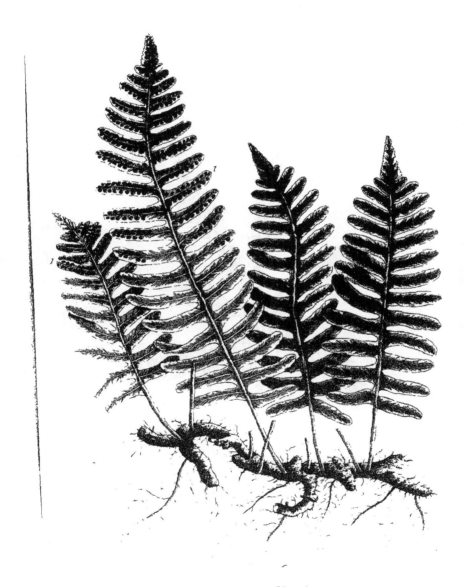

Wall fern or Polypody of the Oak.   Plate   Polypodium Vulgare

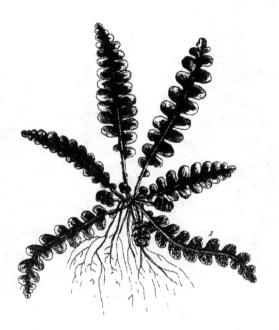

Plate 218

Spleen Wort ceterach Milwast　} a Seed {　Asplenium ceterach ...

56. Blackw. Ill. Edin scabr. Prov.

Plate 217 **Horsetail. Cauda equina**

1 The stalks that bear the Seed grow to be 7 or 8 Inches high & those that bear the Leaves are about 2 Foot high, the Leaves are a bright Green & ÿ Flowers brown
2 It grows in Ditches and marshy Grounds, flowring in March
3 Horsetail is accounted restringent drying & binding, used to stop Bleeding in Wounds, and all Haemorrhages in any part of the Body the catamenia and Fluor albus Ulcerations in ÿ Kidneys or Bladder & is useful in all kinds of Ruptures
4 Greek Ἵππουρις Latin. Equisetum Spanish goda de Mula Italian coda di cavalli French Queve de Cheval German, Roßschwantz Dutch. Paardestaart

Plate 218 *Sea Scurvy-Grass* Cochlearia Britannica marina

1 It grows to be 8 Inches high the Leaves are a light Green & the Flowers white
2 This Scurvy Grass grows in great plenty by the Thames Side below Woolwich and flowers in March and April
3 This Plant is frequently used in Scorbutic Remedies along with the Garden Scurvy Grass, but wanting its fine volatile Parts it seems not so prevalent but abounding more in Saline it may be used to good Purpose as a Diuretic
4 Greek   Latin, Cochlearia Britannica Spanish,   Italian. French Herbe aux Cuilers German   Dutch, Lepelbladen

Plate 219 **White Maiden Hair Adianthum album**

1 The Stalks grow about 3 or 4 Inches high, the Leaves are light Green above and brown underneath by reason of the Seed
2 It grows on old Stone Walls & Buildings
3 This is one of the five Capillary Herbs mentioned in the Dispensatory & has the same Virtues with the rest of the Maiden Hairs, being opening & attenuating and good for Distempers of the Lungs and Breast, and is useful in pectoral Decoctions and Diuretic Apozems
4 Greek Ἀδίαντον λευκόν Latin. Ruta muraria or Salvia Vitae Spanish Culantrillo depozzo blanco Italian Capel Venere bianco French capil Venere blanque German, Frauen Har Dutch Steenruyte

Plate 220 **Black Maiden Hair Adianthum nигrum**

1 This Maiden Hair grows about a Span high the Leaves are a bright Green above and underneath they are covered with small Brown Seed
2 It grows in Shady Lanes and at the Roots of Trees
3 This is also one of the five Capillary Herbs & its Virtues are much the same as ÿ common Maiden Hair being useful for Coughs & all affections of ÿ Lungs and Diseases of ÿ Kidneys, Some commend it as good for the Jaundice
4 Greek Ἀδίαντον μέλον Latin Adianthum nigrum vulgare or Onopteris femina Spanish culantrillo depozzo negro Italian capel venere French capil venere noir German Frauen Har   Dutch Bruinen steenkruyt

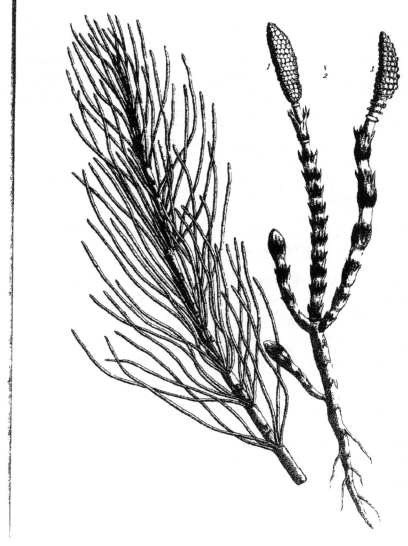

Plate 217

1 *2* *1*

Horsetail   The Head which   Cauda
             contain the Seed

Plate 301

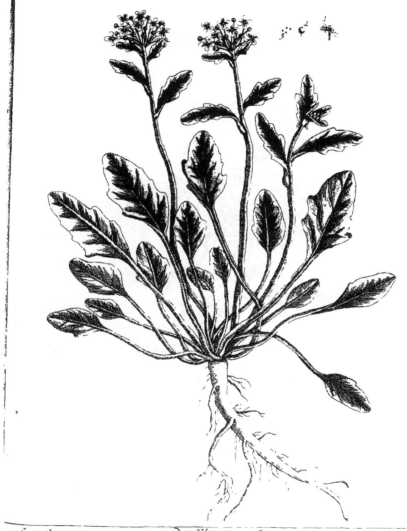

Sea Scurvy grass

Eliz: Blackwell delin: sculp: et Pinx

1 Flower
2 Seed Vessel
3 Seed

Cochlearia Britannica marina

Plate 10

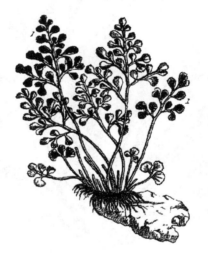

White maiden hair.
English black maidenhair.

The back of
the Leaf.

Adianthum album

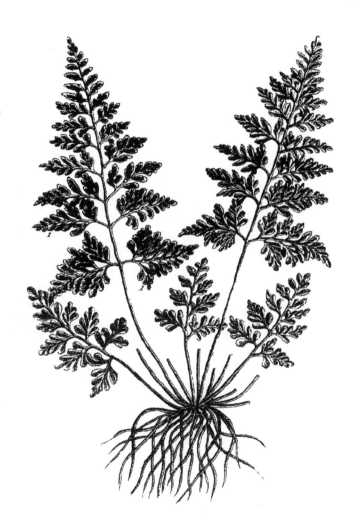

Tab 226

Black Maiden Hair   } 1 The Back of   { Adianthum nigrum
Eliz Blackwell delin Sculp et Pinx { the Leaf   {

Plate 221 *The East India Tamarind Tamarindus indica Orientalis.*

1 This Tree differs from the West India Tamarind in the Leaves & Fruit & is better to be used in Medicines than the other because the Fruit contains more Pulp

2 It grows in the East Indies and flowers in the Spring this Specimen of the Tree and fruit is taken from the Malabar Garden

3 Tamarinds are accounted cooling and opening good to purge choleric Humors and correct the bilious Heat of the Stomach and Bowels they also are good to allay Thirst, promote Urine and help the Jaundice

4 Greek, Ὀξυφοίνικες Latin, Tamarindi Spanish Italian French. German. Dutch,

---

Plate 222 *Butterbur. Petasites.*

1 The Stalks grow about a Span high, the Leaves are a bright Green above and whitish underneath, and the Flowers purplish

2 It grows in Marshy Grounds, and on Banks by River Sides & flowers the Beginning of March

3 The Roots are esteem'd sudorific and alexipharmic good for all Kinds of Fevers and malignant Distempers, preventing Fainting and shortness of Breath provoking Urine and destroying joint Worms Outwardly they are used as a Cataplasm for pestilential Buboes and Plague Sores A good Quantity of them is put into the Ag Theriaculis

4 Greek, Βήχιον μέγα Latin Petasites major Spanish. Italian, Farfara maggiore French. German. Pestilenzwurt Dutch

---

Plate 223 *Ladie's Smock, Cuckowflower Cardamine*

1 The Stalks grow about a Foot high, the Leaves are a grass Green and the Flowers a pale purple, and often white

2 It grows in Meadows and on Banks flowring in March and April

3 It is accounted heating and warming good for the Scurvy, the Stone and Gravel, Dropsy and Jaundice

4 Greek, Σισύμβριον ἕτερον Latin Nasturtium pratense magno flore Spanish Berros Italian Cressione minore French. Gession de l'Eau German, Wasser Gressen Dutch.

Plate 224 *Wild Naven Napus sylvestris.*

1 The Stalks grow to be a Foot high, the Leaves are a bright Green, and the Flowers yellow

2 It grows on Banks and the Edges of Fields flowring in April

3 The Ancients commend the Seed as good against all Kinds of Poisons and the Bites of venemous Creatures, and good to provoke Urine and the Terms Andromachus junior prefers the Seed of this Wild sort before the garden as of a hotter Nature

Greek Βουνία ἀγρια Latin Bunias sylvestris Spanish Italian Navone salvatico French. Navet sauvage German. Stechrüben Dutch

No 56

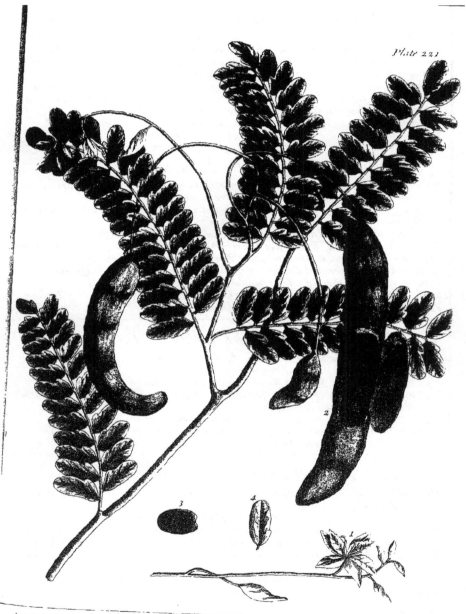

Plate 221

East Indie Tamarind
Tamarindus indica

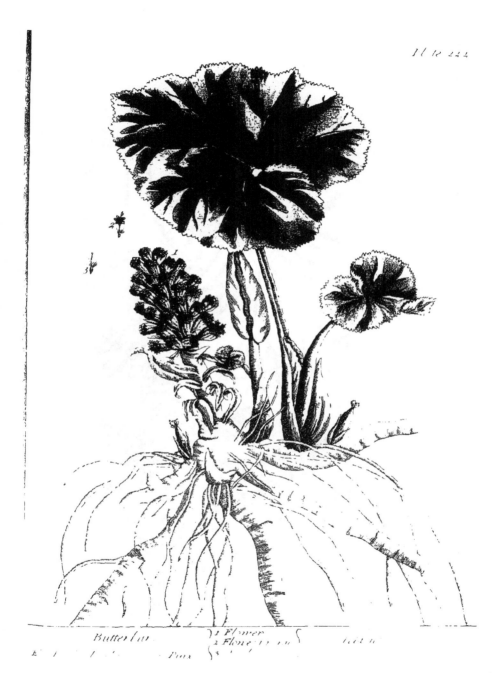

Butterbur   1 Flower
                 2 Flower

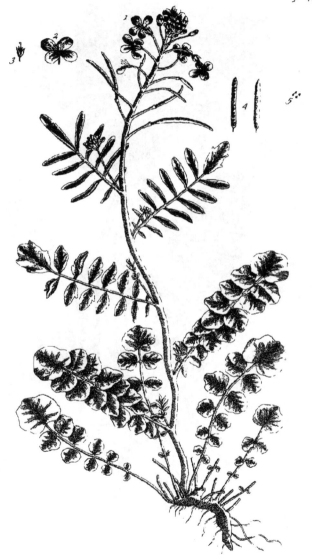

Pl. 112. 2.

Ladies Smock   Cardamine

Elz Ph.

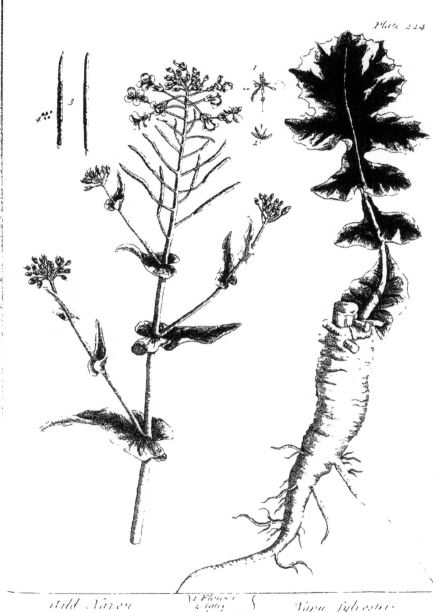

Plate 224

Wild Navew   1 Flower   Napu Sylvestris
                              2 ....
                              3 Seed .....

Plate 225 Ground Ivy or Alehoof Hedera terrestris

1 The Stalks grow about eight Inches long the Leaves are a grass Green
and the Flowers blue
2 It grows by Hedges and Banks flowring in April
3 This Plant is esteem'd a very good Pectoral, being much used for Coughs
Shortness of Breath and other Disorders of the Lungs, for which a Tea made
of the Leaves & a Syrup of the Juice is very beneficial It is this Plant that
they make the Gill Ale with, being accounted antiscorbutic and apperative and
good to provoke Urine & cleanse ÿ Ureters Some Authors commend it steeped
in Brandy as of Great Service against the Collic The Officinal Preparation
is the Syrup of ÿ Juice
4 Greek. Κιαρὸς χεϱοαῖ@ Latin, Chamaecissus Spanish, Eda Italian Hedera
terrestris French. Lierre de la Terre German Gundelreben. Dutch Hondsdraf

Plate 226 The Cowslip or Paigle Paralysis

1 The Stalks grow about six Inches high, the Leaves are a grass Green above
and whitish underneath, and the Flowers yellow
2 It grows in moist Meadows and Marshes, flowring in April
3 The Flowers are accounted cordial, and beneficial to the nervous Sistem
good against the Epilepsy Palsy Apoplexy & Pains in ÿ Head Some say they
are anodyne & good to procure Sleep for which Purpose they make Tea of them
The Leaves are used in warming, strengthening Ointments, particularly the
Unguent Nervinum Officinal Preparations are The Simple Water The
Syrup and the Conserve
4 Greek.   Latin, Primula veris major Spanish,   Italian
Fiore di Primavera. French. Primvere German Schlusselblumen Dutch Sleutelblom

Plate 227 Scurvy-Grass Cochlearia Batava

1 The Stalks grow to be eight or nine Inches high, the Leaves are a grass
Green and the Flowers white
2 It grows wild in the North of England by the Sea Side but is very much cultivated
in Gardens, and flowers in April
3 This Plant abounds with fine volatile Parts and therefore ÿ Herb infused or the
Juice express'd is more prevalent than a Decoction the volatile Part flying away
in the Boiling and is accounted a Specific Remedy against the Scurvy Cleansing
and purifying the Juices of the Body from the bad Effects of that Distemper and
clearing the Skin from Scabs Pimples & foul Eruptions Officinal Preparations
are The Simple Water The Spirit and a Conserve
4 Greek.   Latin Cochlearia Batava rotundifolia hortensis Spanish
Italian,   French.   German. Loffelcraut Dutch Tepelbladen

Plate 228 Wake Robin or Cuckow-pint Arum

1 The Stalks grow more than a Foot & an half high the Leaves are a deep Green
the Flowers purple and the Fruit a yellowish Red
2 It grows in Hedges and dry Ditches and flowers in May
3 The Roots tryed & powdered are accounted good for a tachexy the Scurvy & Isthma
and the Quantity of a Drachm of ÿ Roots of ÿ Spotted sort dryed is commended as an excel
lent Antipestilential & if Leaves beat to a cataplasm is good for Plague Sores Matthiolus says a
Poultice of ÿ Roots beat to mash & mix'd with cow Dung eases the Pains of the Gout
4 Greek Άρον Latin Arum maculatum Mando uuris Spanish Uno, Italian,
Gigaro French. Iit de chien terreau Dutch her ember Dutch Kalfsvoet

Plate 215

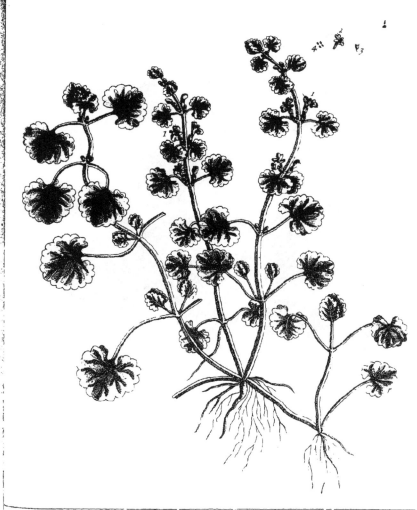

Ground Ivy or Alehoof

Hedera terrestris.

Plate 226

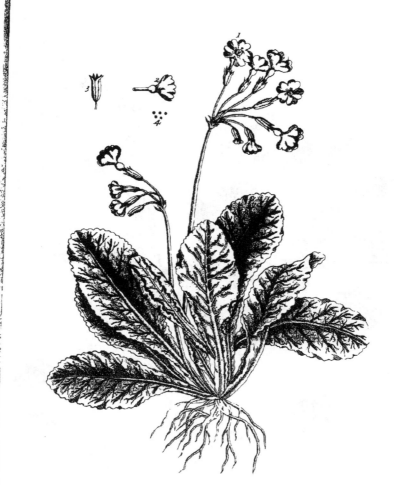

The Cowslip or Paigle

Eliz. Blackwell delin. sculp et Pinx.

1 Flower
2 Flower open aa
3 Calix
4 Seed

Paralysis

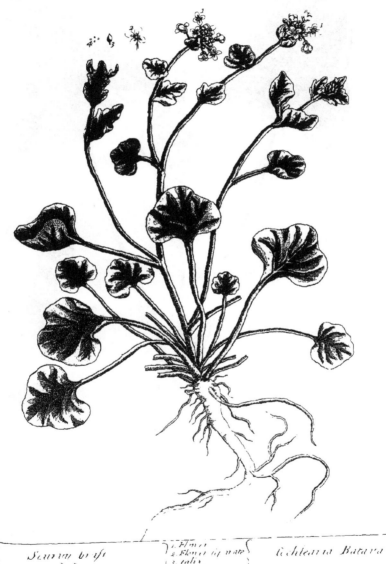

Scurvy grass

Eliz Blackwell delin et sculp

1. Flower
2. Flower _____
3. tube
4. seed

Cochlearia Batava

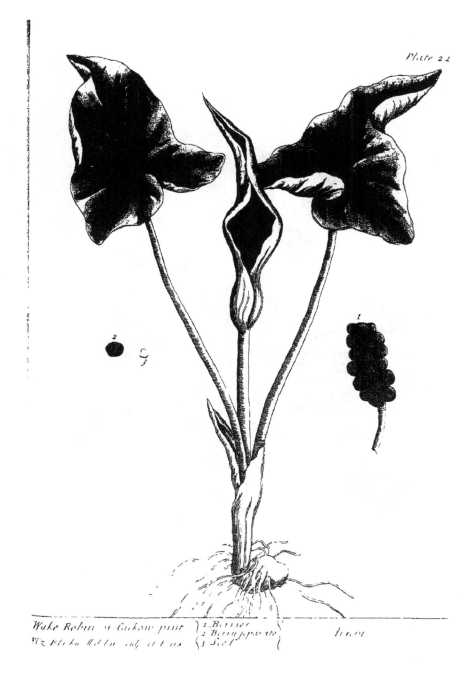

Plate 22

2

3

1

Wake Robin a Cuckow pint {1. Berries
Flz Flicha Wilden only et l'air {2. Benyspante
{3. Seed   hom

Plate 229 The Common Aloes Aloe vulgaris

1 The Stalks grow about two or three Foot high, the Leaves are a hutish
Green, and the Flowers a pale yellow

2 It grows in Spain Italy and the West Indies flowring in the Spring

3 The Aloes Hepatica of the Shops or the Barbadoes Aloes is made from this Plant
Aloes is a purging Medicine much in Use and very beneficial to cold moist
Constitutions, but is seldom given by it self unless it be to Children for ye Worms
It is a main Ingredient in most of the Officinal Pills, as also in ye Species Hiera Picra

4 Greek Αλόη Latin Aloe Spanish Hierva babosa Italian Aloe French Aloes
German Bitter Aloes Dutch Aloe

Plate 230 Sorrel Acetosa

1 The Stalks grow eight or ten Inches high, the Leaves are a grass Green,
and the Flowers small and Staminous

2 It grows in Fields and Meadows, flowring in May

3 The Leaves are accounted cooling and cordial and very good in Fevers
resisting Putrefaction The Root is esteem'd serviceable in the Scurvy & bilious
Fluxes The Seed is restringent, & is put into Diascordium & other binding Medicines

4 Greek Οξαλις Latin Oxalis & Acetosa pratensis Spanish Azedas Italian
Acetosa French Saliette German Sawr Umpffer Dutch Veld Suringh

Plate 231 Turnep Rapum.

1 The Stalks grow about three Foot high, the Leaves are a grass Green
and the Flowers yellow

2 It is sown in Fields and Gardens flowring in April

3 Turneps are accounted very wholesome and nourishing, but somewhat windy
A Syrup made with slices of Turnep and brown Sugar Candy baked in an
Oven, is commended as a good pectoral and of great Service for Coughs
and Consumptions

4 Greek Γογγυλη Latin Rapum Spanish Nabo Italian Rapo French Rave
German Ruben, Dutch, Raapen knollen

Plate 232 Wall-pepper or Stonecrop Sedum minimum

1 The Stalks grow about five Inches high, the Leaves are a pale Green
and the Flowers yellow

2 It grows on Walls and Houses flowring in May

3 This Plant is often used in the Shops for the Sedum minus by the Ignorance
of the Herb Women, altho its Qualities are directly opposite to the other Sedums
and is more apt to raise than cure Inflammations The Stonecrop is much
commended for the Scurvy and King's Evil taken inwardly in Decoctions
and the Limbs bathed with it in Fomentations

Greek Αειζωον μικρον Latin Sempervivum minimum Spanish
Semperviva Italian Herba Grassella French Joubarbe le plus petit
German Rawer Pfeffer Dutch Maus Peper

No 58

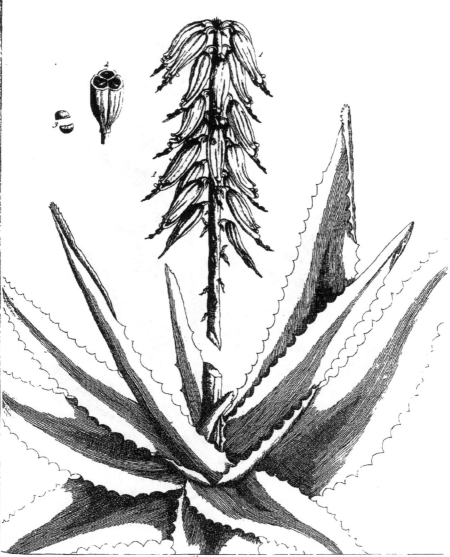

Plate 228

The Common Aloes

Eliz Blackwell delin: sculp: et Pinx:

1 Flower
2 Seed Vessel open'd
3 Seed

Aloe vulgaris

Plate

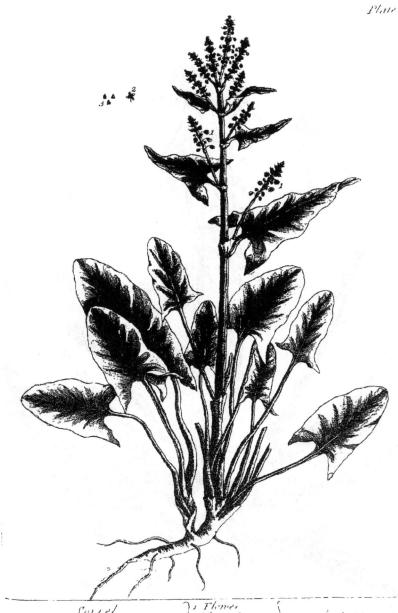

Sorrel

Fl. Blackwell . . . Pin.

1 Flower
2 Flower bud
3 Seed

Plate 231

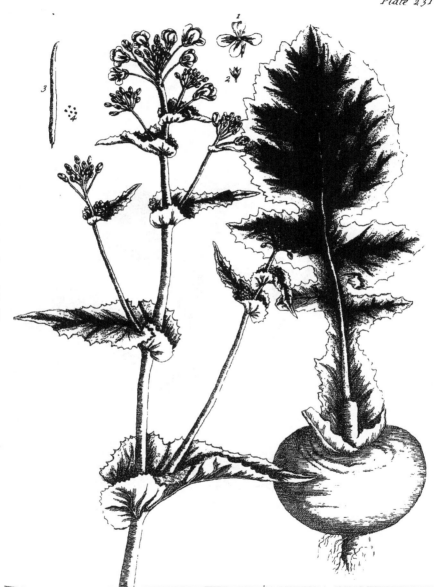

Turnep

Eliz: Blackwell delin: sculp et pinx

1 Flower
2 Calax
3 Pod
4 Seed

Rapum

Plate 1

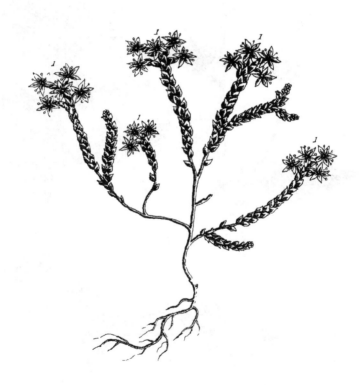

Wall-pepper or Stonecrop
Eliz Blackwell delineavit sculpsit Pinx } 1 Flower { Sedum vermium

Plate 23, Yellow Asphodel Kingspear Asphodelus luteus &c &c Royal
the stalks grow about one Foot high the Leaves are a dark blue green tiped with
a ... green and the Flowers yellow

It grows naturally in Italy and Sicily and is planted here in Gardens flowrs
in ... April and May

Dioscorides commends the Root as good to provoke Urine and brings down the
Water and an Ointment made from the Ashes of the Root he says procures
the Hair to grow when it has fallen off thro' any Distemper

Greek Ασφοδελος luteus or μαλιους Latin Asphodelus foemina or luteus
Spanish Gamones Italian Anpodillo French. Sifodele German Gelb
Affodellwurk, Dutch.

Plate 224 *Wild Bugloss Buglossum Sylvestre*
The Stalks grow near a Foot high the Leaves are a babe grass Green
and the Flowers a light Blue

It grows by Hedges and amongst Corn flowring in April and May

Bugloss is much of the Nature of Borrage being accounted cordial and
good to exhilarate the Spirits & drive away Melancholy & is of Service
in hypocondriac and hysteric Disorders

Greek Βουγλωσσον αγριον Latin Buglossum sylvestre minus Spanish
Borrajenes Italian Buglossa salvatica French Buglose sauvage German
Ochsenzung Dutch Buglosse or Ossetongen

Plate 225 *Red Beet Beta rubra in minor*
The stalk grow about two Foot high the Leaves a ... dark Green tinctured
with Purple and the Flowers small and Stamina

It is planted in Gardens and flowers in April and May

Beet are esteemd good to loosen the Belly and temperate hot choleric Humors
the Juice of y' Root is sometimes used as an Errhine being snuffed up y' ...
to clear the Head of Flegm and mucous Humors and by that means to
help old Head achs

Greek Τευτλον ερυθρος Latin Beta rubra vulgaris Spanish Azelgas Italian
Bietola rossa French Ponee rouge German Rot Ruben Dutch Roode Beet

---

Plate 226 *Chervil Chaerefolium*
The Stalks grow about a Foot high the Leaves are a grass Green
and the Flowers white

It is sown in Gardens flowring in April and May

This Plant has much of the nature of Parsley being aperitive & attenuating
and good for the Stone and Gravel and to provoke Urine and the Menses

Greek Χαιρεφυλλον Latin Chaerophyllum sativum Spanish
Italian Cerpoglio French   German Gerbelkraut Dutch Kervel

A. 50

Plate 233

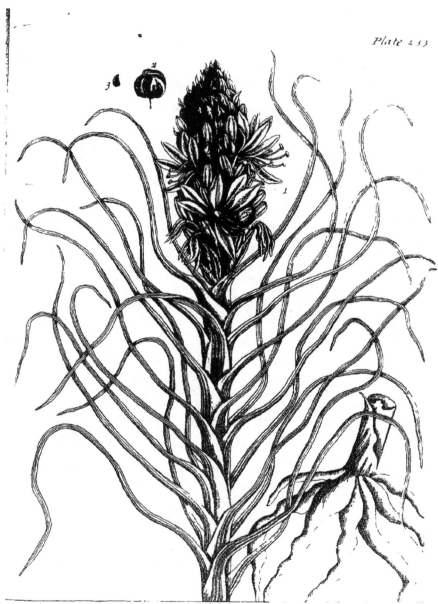

Yellow Asphodel or Kinas Spear Flower

Eliz Blackwell delin sculp et Pinx

Plate 234

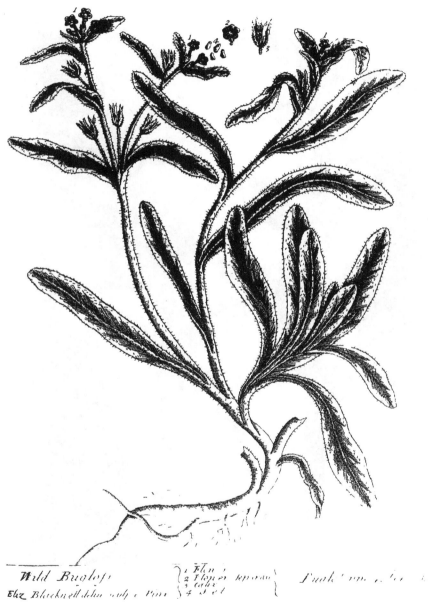

Wild Buglofs

Eliz Blackwell delin: sculp: et Pinx:

1 Flos
2 Flores separaui
3 Calix
4 Sel

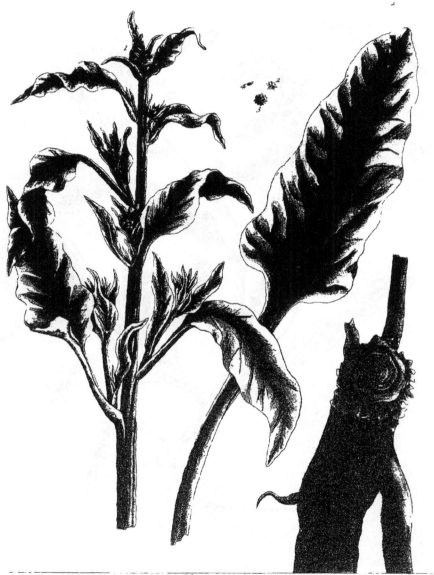

Plate 255.

Red Beet.

1 Flower
2 Flower Magnified
3 ...
4 Seed.

Beta rubra or nigra

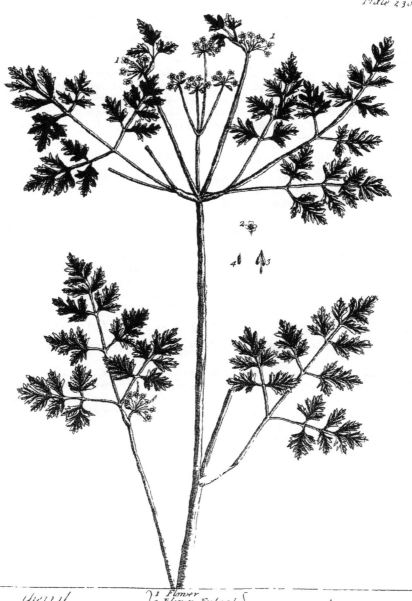

Plate 230

Chervil

Th . . . .

1 Flower
2 Flower Enlarged
3 Seed Vessel open
4 . . .

Chae. of olium.

Plate 237 *Fumitory Fumaria*

The Stalks grow about eight Inches high the Leaves are a light Green
and the Flowers Purple

It grows in Fields and till'd Grounds flowring in May

This Plant is accounted a great Cleanser of the Blood being good for all Sorts of
Cutaneous Distempers & leprous Disorders It is much drank with Whey in the
Spring to purge & purify y Blood & help y Scurvy Jaundice & Affections of the Spleen

Greek Καπνὸς Latin Fumaria officinarum et Dioscoridis Spanish Palomelha Italian
Fumosterno French Fumeterre German, Erdrauch Rakentorbel Dutch Duyderkerdel

---

Plate 238 *The true white Asphodel Asphodelus verus, albus*

The Stalks grow about three Foot high, the Leaves are a light grass Green and
the Flowers white with purple Veins

It is a native of Spain, Italy and the Southern Parts of France and is planted
here in Gardens flowring in April

Dioscorides commends the Root as good for eating Ulcers Inflammations in the
Breast or Blotches in the Skin The Juice of the Root he says cures Scabby Ears
and eases the Pain of the Teeth by pouring some of it into y contrary Ear where
the Tooth aches He also recommends y Root to provoke Urine & bring down the Menses

Greek, Ασφόδελος Latin, Asphodelus albus ramosus mas Spanish Gamones
Italian, Anfodillo French, Asfodele German. Affodilwurt Dutch.

Plate 239 *Great Woolfs-bane or Leopard's bane Doronicum Romanorum*

The Stalks grow about eighteen Inches high, the Leaves are a dull Green and
the Flowers yellow

It is a native of the Alps and is planted here in Gardens flowring in April

Some commend the Root against the Poison of Scorpions others account it a
Poison and say it will destroy Woolves, Dogs & other Animals Those who have
a mind to see y Arguments on both Sides may consult Lobel & Matthiolus

Greek. Latin, Doronicum salu Scorpio Spanish.
Italian, Doronico French, Le Doronic German gemsenwurt Dutch Doronicum

---

Plate 240 *Birch Betula*

This grows to be a tall Tree the Leaves are a bright grass Green
and the Catkins brownish

It grows in Woods and the Catkins come out in April

The Liquor that comes from this Tree tored in the Spring is accounted
good for the Stone Gravel Stranguary & bloody Urine The Leaves are often
good for the Dropsy & Itch used both inwardly & outwardly The Wood inest to
Juniper is preferd to burn in times of Pestilence & contagious Distempers

Greek Σημύδα Latin Betula Spanish   Italian Betula French
Le Bouleau German Bircken Dutch.

No 60

Plate 43.

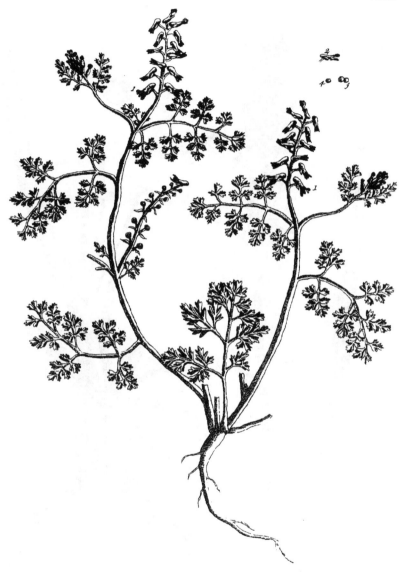

Fumitory

1 Flower
2 Flower separate
3 Seed Vessel open
4 Seed

Fumaria

Eliz Blackwell delin. Scul et Pinx

Plate 498

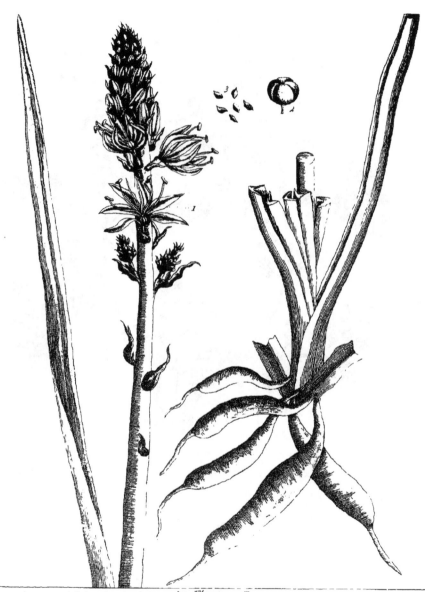

The true white Asphodel

Eliz. Blackwell delin. sculp et Pinx

1 Flower
2 Seed Vessel
3 Seed

Asphodelus verus albus

Plate 254

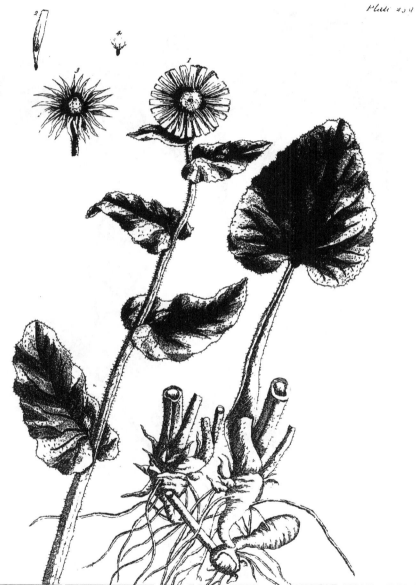

Great Wolfsbane or Leopards bane
the Blasd Ilian . . .

1 Flower
2 Flower separate
3 . . .

Doronicum Romanorum

Plate 240

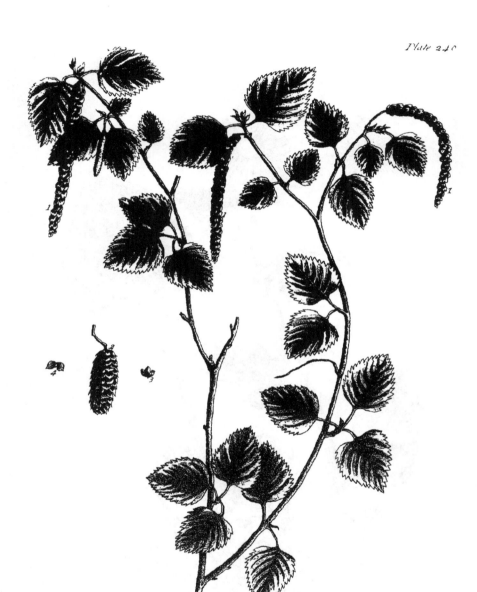

Birch

viz Blackwell delin. culp. et Pinx

1 catkin
2 cone
3 Scale of the cone
4 Scale with y Seed

Betula

Plate 241 Stechas, or French Lavender Stœchas arabica ~ purpurea

1 This Shrub grows about three Foot high the Leaves are a whitish Green and the Flowers a deep Purple

2 It grows naturally in Spain and the Southern Parts of France and is planted here in Gardens, flowring in April and May

3 The Flowers are accounted cordial & cephalic Strengthening the genus Nervosum and are usefull in Apoplexies Palsies & Convulsions They are also opening & attenuating promoting the Catamenia and resisting Poisons

4 Greek, Στιχας or Στοιχάς Latin Stœchas arabica or Stœchas purpurea Spanish Tomani or Cantuello Italian, Stechade French. Stœchados German Stuhaskraut Dutch, Stœchas

---

Plate 242 Rocket Eruca

1 The Stalks grow about three Foot high, the Leaves are a grass Green and the Flowers white with purple Veins

2 It is sown in Gardens, and flowers in April and May

3 The Leaves are often eat as a Sallad with other Herbs Some account it a Stimulus to Venery, & a good Diuretic Matthiolus commends the Syrup of the Leaves as good for Childrens Coughs Cammerarius that an equal Part of Rocket and Cummin Seed powdred is a good Preservative against the Apoplexy

4 Greek, Ευζομον Latin, Eruca latifolia alba Spanish, Oruga Italian, Ruccla French, Roquette German Beiss Senff Dutch Rakette

---

Plate 243 Sweet-Cicely Myrrhis

1 The Stalks grow about four Foot high, the Leaves are a bright grass Green and the Flowers white

2 It is sown in Gardens and flowers in April and May

3 This Plant is often eat as a Sallad being much of the same Nature as Chervil consisting of hot & thin Parts being good for cold windy Stomachs, opening Obstructions of the Liver and Spleen, & provoking Urine

Greek, Μύρρις Latin, Myrrhis major & Cicutaria odorata Spanish Italian, Mirrade French. German, Belscher Corbel Dutch

---

Plate 244 Broom Genista

The Stalks grow about Eight or ten Foot high the Leaves are a dark Green and the Flowers a bright Yellow

It grows in Fields and on Commons, flowring in May

The Stalks Flowers & Seed are used & are esteem'd good to provoke Urine & open Obstructions of the Liver & Spleen It is esteem'd good for a Dropsy infused in common Drink or it selfe infused in Wine causing great Discharges of Water to them Some pickle its Flowers before they are full blown with Salt & Vineagr and use them instead of Capers esteeming them good against Diseases of the Liver & Spleen

Greek   Latin Genista angulosa et Scoparia Spanish Geniesta Italian Ginestra French.   German, Ginst Dutch Brem

No 61

Plate 241

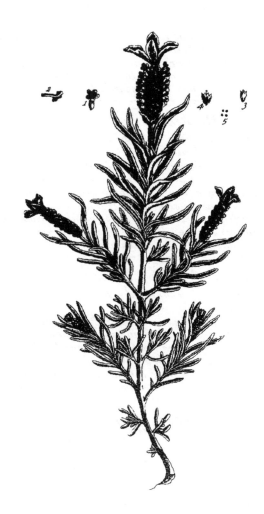

Stechas or French Lavender
Eliz Blackwell delin sculp et Pinx

1 Flower
2 Flower separate
3 Calix
4 Calix open
5 Seed

Stoechas arabica or purpurea

Plate 242

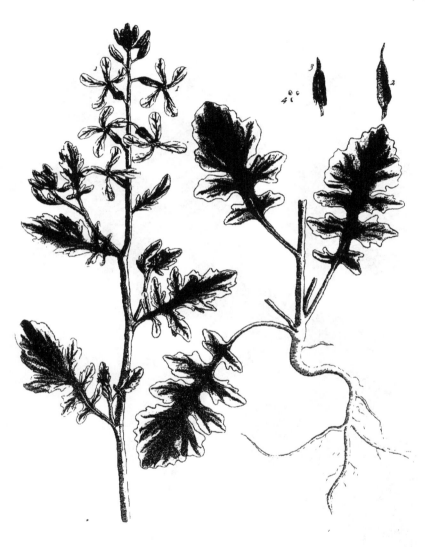

Rocket   1 Flower   Eruca
             2 Seed Vessel
             3 Seed Vessel open
Blackw. Delin. Sculp. Pinx   4 Seed

Plate 243

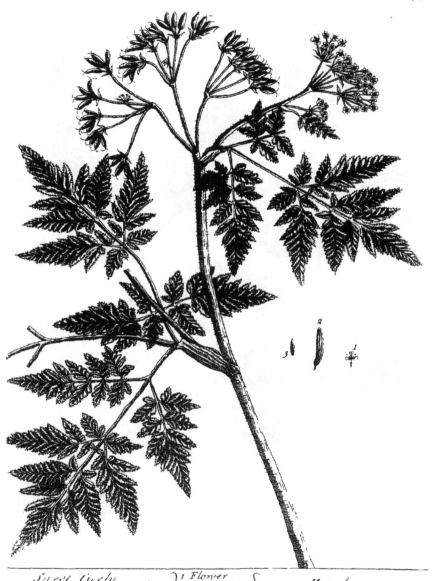

Sweet Cicely   1 *Flower*
              2 *Seed Vessel*
              3 *Seed*   *Myrrhis*

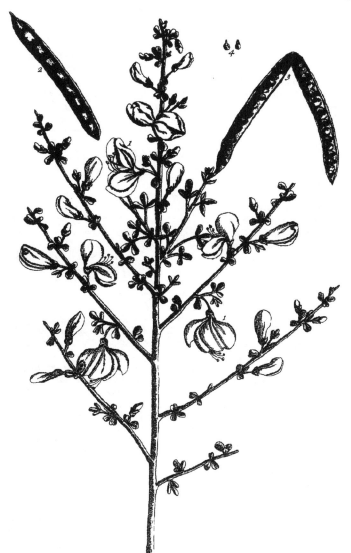

Plate 244

Broom

Mr. Birkn Hd low mdp e Cure.

1 Flower
2 Pod
3 Pod y en
4 Seed

Genista

Plate 245 Male Piony Paeonia mas

1 The Stalk grow about one Foot high the Leaves are a dark gray green with reddish Veins and the Flowers red
2 It is planted in Gardens and flowers in April and May
3 The Flowers Seed & Roots are esteemed cephalic & good for the Epilepsy Apoplexy & all kinds of Convulsions both in young & old They are also accounted good in hysteric Cases, Obstructions of the Menses and the Retention of the Lochia The Root and Seed are hung about Childrens Necks to prevent Convulsions in Breeding their Teeth
4 Greek Γ...... idn or Παιονία Latin Paeonia folio nigricante splendido que Mas Spanish Rosa del Monte Italian Peonia French Pivoine or Pyvoine German Peonien Dutch Pioene maneke

Plate 246 Woad Isatis.

1 The Stalks grow about three or four Foot high the Leaves are a willow Green and the Flowers yellow
2 It grows wild in several Parts of England but is generally Sown for the Use of the Dyers and flowers in May
3 Woad is esteemd restringent & drying and is good to stop inward & outward Bleedings Some commend it much for Ruptures & Strains and to strengthen the Joints It is an Ingredient in the Emplastrum ad Herniam
4 Greek Ισάτι Latin Glastum & Isatis sativa or latifolia Spanish, Pastel Italian Guado French Gueda or Pastel German Weid Dutch.

Plate 247 The Wallnut Juglans

1 This grows to be a large Tree the Leaves are a yellow Green & ÿ Catkins yellowish
2 It is planted in Walks Parks & Fields, and the Catkins come out in April
3 The Bark is accounted a strong Emetic either Green or dried and powdered The Green Nuts are cordial & alexipharmic being of great Use in all contagious malignant Distempers & even the Plague they are one of the Principal Ingredients in the Treacle Water The Nuts preserved are good to be eat in a Morning to prevent Infection in the time of Pestilential Distempers Two or three Ounces of the Oil expressd from the ripe Kernels is a very good Medicine for the Stone and Gravel The Shells powdered or burnt are accounted restringent
4 Greek Κάρυα Βασιλικὰ Latin Nux juglans or regia vulgaris Spanish Noces Italian Noce French Noix German Welschnuss Dutch Ockernooten

Plate 248 Black Poplar Populus nigra

1 It grows to be a large Tree the Leaves are a bright grass Green the Catkins yellowish and the Berries Green
2 It grows by Watery Places and Rivers and the Catkins come out in April The Leaves & Buds are used to make ÿ Unguentum Populeon Schroder says the Women in Germany used Buds to make their Hair grow thick & ornamental
4 Greek Γ...... Latin Populus nigra Spanish Alamo nianialio Italian Pople nero French Tremble German Aspen or Popel Weiden Dutch Swarte Populier

No 62

Plate 245

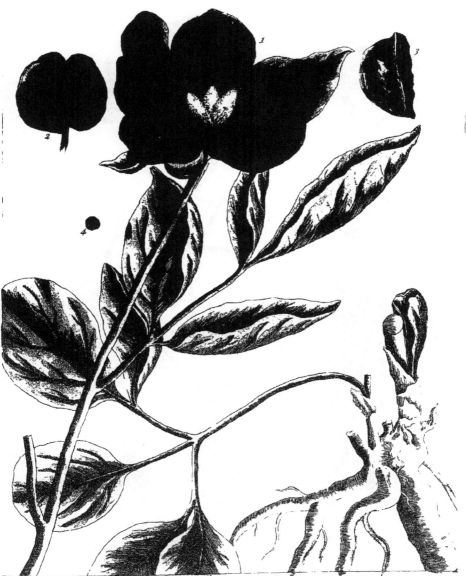

Male Piony

1. Flower
2. Seed Vessel
3. Seed vessel open
4. Seed

Freonia mas

Eliz Blackwell delin sculp. et Pinx

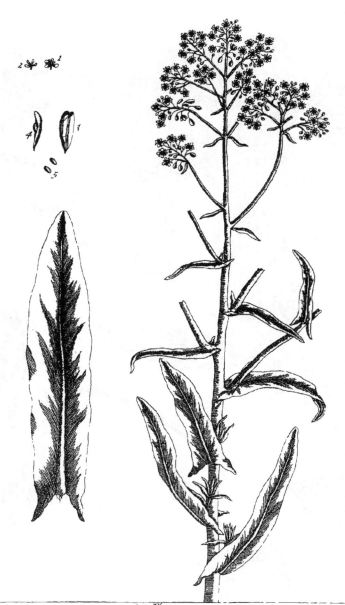

Plate 246

Head

Viz. Black noll John only or Pine

1 Flower
2. dales
3. stalk with open
4. Seed head open
5. seed

Gratis

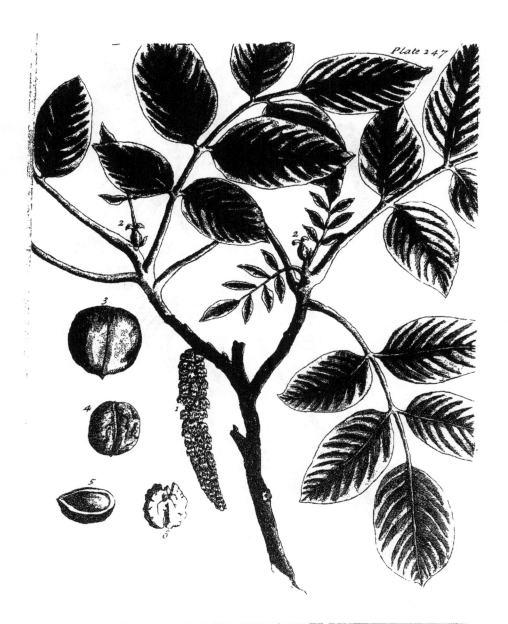

Plate 247

The Wallnut   1 catkin   4 Shel
                2 Flower   5 Shel open   Juglan
Eliz Blackwell delin. ... nula et Pinx   3 Green Nut   6 Seed

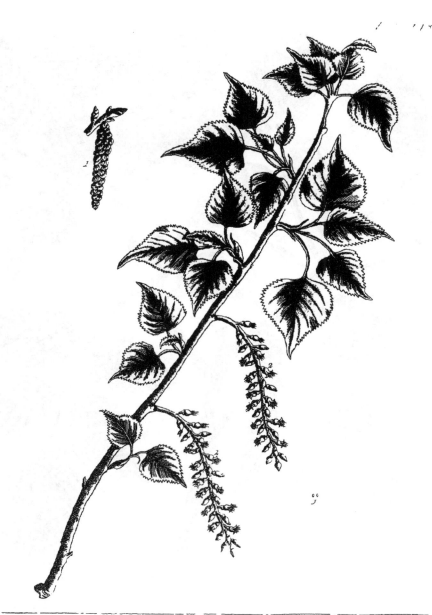

Black Poplar
The Blackwell delineaunt et Pinx

1 Catkin
4 Fruit
3 Seed

Populus nigra

Plate 249 Hounds-tongue *Cynoglossum*

1 The stalks grow two or three Foot high the Leaves are a blue Green, and the Flowers red

2 It grows by Hedges and the sides of Roads flowring in May & June

3 The Root is accounted cold drying & binding good for Catarrhous Defluxions upon the Lungs, and all kinds of Fluxes & Haemorrhagies & a Gonorrhea Some account it a vulnerary & use it for scrophulous Tumors, taken inwardly or applied outwardly as a cataplasm The Officinal Preparation is of Pilul Cynogloss

4 Greek Κυνόγλωσσον Latin Cynoglossa & Cynoglossum majus vulgare Spanish Italian Lengua canina French Langue de Chien German Hundstung Dutch Hondstonge

---

Plate 250 Valerian *Valeriana* or *Phu*.

1 The stalks grow three Foot high, the Leaves are a grass Green and the Flowers white

2 It is a Native of Italy and is planted here in Gardens flowring in May

3 The Root is esteem'd alexipharmic sudorific & Cephalic being of great Service in malignant Fevers & pestilential Distempers It also helps the Head & Nerves provokes Urine and brings down the Menses It is an Ingredient in the Theriaca and Mithridate

4 Greek Φοῦ & Ἀσία Ναάδος Latin Valeriana hortensis & Phu folio Olusatri Dioscoridis Spanish Yerva benedicta Italian Valeriana French Valerienne German Valdrian Dutch Hof Valeriana

---

Plate 251 Solomon's-Seal *Polygonatum* & *Sigillum Solomonis*

1 The stalks grow two Foot high the Leaves are a grass Green above and a yellow Green underneath and the Flowers white tinctured with Green

2 It grows wild in several Woods & Copses here and flowers in May

3 The Leaves & Root are used being esteem'd vulnerary and restringent good to stop all Kinds of Fluxes & Haemorrhagies & consolidate Wounds Fractures & Ruptures, especially the Root Matthiolus commends the Root preserved in Sugar as of great Service against ÿ Fluor albus Some say a cataplasm of ÿ Root is good to take away black & blue Marks arising from Contusions

4 Greek Πολυγόνατον Latin Polygonatum latifolium vulgare Spanish, Italian Ginocchietto French Geniculiere German Weiss Wurt Dutch Salomons Segel

---

Plate 252 Comfrey *Symphytum* & *Consolida major*

1 The stalks grow 3 Foot high the Leaves are a dull grass Green & ÿ Flowers white

2 It grows on Banks by River sides & Watery Places flowring in May & June

3 The Root Leaves & Flowers are used being accounted vulnerary whence it takes the Name of Consolida It is esteem'd good for inward Bruises spitting of Blood and sharp corroding Humours that cause Erosions in the Bowels Some commend the Root beat to a cataplasm as good for the Gout The Officinal Preparation is the Syrup de Symphyto

4 Greek Σύμφυτον & σος Latin Consolida major Spanish Consuelda major Italian Consolida maggiore French Oreille de ane German Schwartzwurt Dutch Smeerwortel

Nᵉ 03

Plate 149

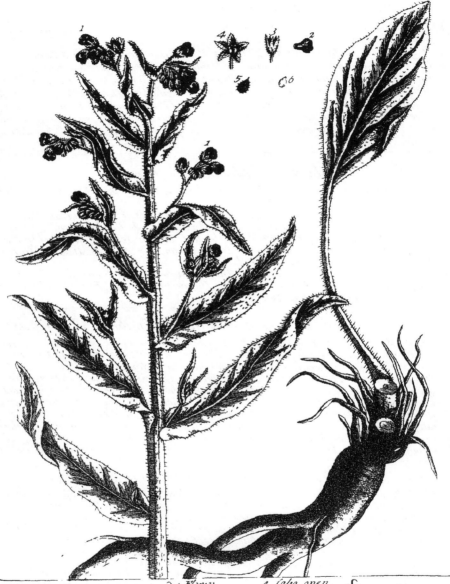

Hounds-tonaue

Eliz Blackwell delin sculp et Pinx

1 Flower
2 Flower separate
3 Color
4 Calix open
5 Shel of ü Seed
6 Seed

{ *Cunoalossum*

Plate 250

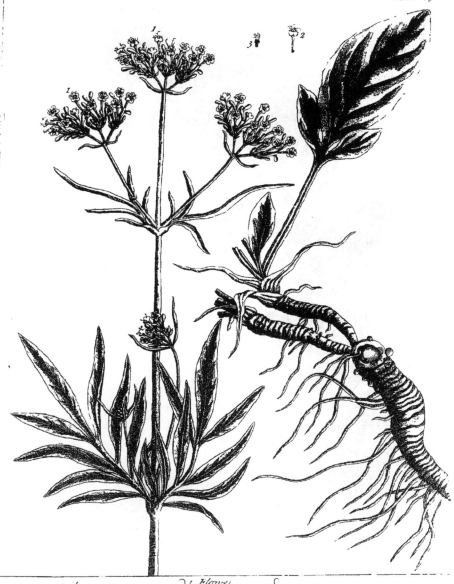

Valerian

Eh-in knell ahn nah... Phu

1 Flower
2 Flower separate
3 Seed

Valeriana . Phu

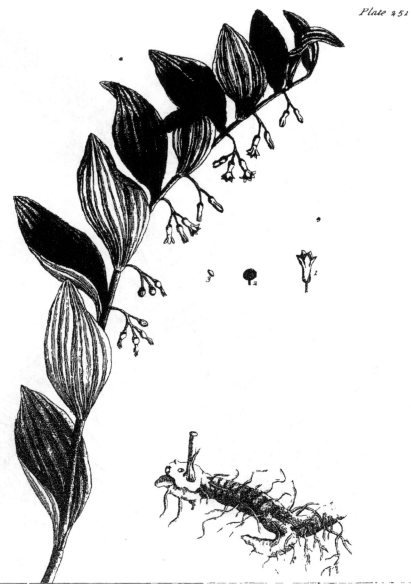

Plate 251

Solomon's Seal

Fl: Blackwell del. bu culp. et Sinx

Flower
Root

Polygonatum & Sigillum Solomonis

Plate 252

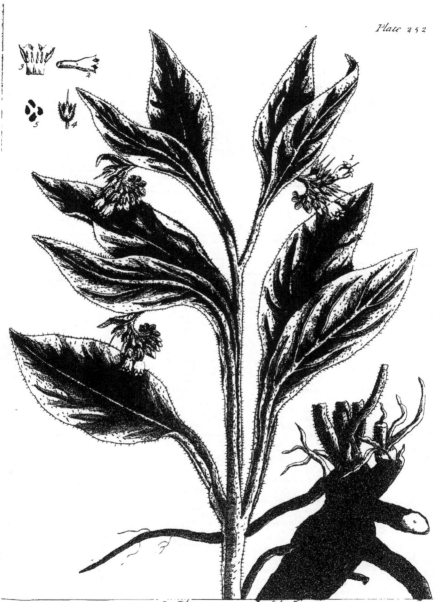

Comfrey

Fliz Blackn ll delin sculp et Pinx

1 Flower
2 Flower separate
3 Flower open

4 Calix
5 Seed

Symphytum &
consolida major